Intimacy Unbound:

"The Secret to Alluring Intelligence"

I0704442

By

Diane T. Wee

About the Author

Diane T. Wee is a well-known psychotherapist and relationship expert who has received international recognition for her research on the intricacies of human relationships. She is fluent in nine languages and has a thorough awareness of cultural dynamics, which she applies to her work. Diane T. Wee has been practicing couples therapy for almost three decades, specializing in the subtle dance of love and desire. She is noted for her bold and perceptive views on intimacy, sexuality, and the issues that modern couples face. Her method is distinguished by a balance of realism and optimism, with the goal of assisting people in cultivating lively and durable relationships. Diane is also the author of "THE POWER OF EMPATHY: A GUIDE TO COMPASSIONATE CONNECTIONS." Her novels have been translated into various languages, demonstrating her wide appeal and the universality of her thoughts.

Table of Contents

Chapter 8:When Love Meets Desire:
Maintaining Sexual Chemistry Over Time
Strategies for Rekindling Passion

Chapter 9:Cultural Influences on Sexuality
How Society Shapes Our Desires
Breaking Free from Normative Expectations

Chapter 10:Conclusion: The Art of Keeping Desire Alive
Embracing the Ongoing Journey
The Future of Intimacy and Eroticism

Chapter 1:Introduction: The Paradox of Love and Desire

The interaction of love and desire is a conundrum that many people find fascinating and challenging. Love thrives on intimacy, stability, and familiarity, but desire thrives on distance, mystery, and the unknown. This dichotomy provides an intriguing tension: how can we balance both in long-term relationships?

Erotic intelligence is the ability to harmonize seemingly contradictory forces. It entails comprehending the nature of desire, appreciating its significance in a loving relationship, and actively fostering it despite the inherent paradoxes. Erotic intelligence is more than just sexual skills or prowess; it is about sustaining a sense of wonder, playfulness, and connection that fuels passion.

The Function of Vulnerability in Desire
Desire is profoundly linked to vulnerability. To desire someone and be desired in return necessitates disclosing parts of oneself that are frequently hidden. This vulnerability can be both exciting and terrible. In the safety of a committed relationship, it is tempting to protect oneself from vulnerability in order to avoid rejection or pain. However, this protective instinct might suppress desire.

When partners allow themselves to be vulnerable with one another, they create a space for deeper intimacy and connection. Vulnerability encourages honesty, creating an environment in which both partners feel recognized and appreciated for who they truly are. This acceptance creates a safe environment in which couples can explore their dreams and wants without fear of being judged.

The Effect of Routine on Desire
Long-term relationships can suffer from a lack of desire due to routine. Routines provide stability and predictability, which are key components of a loving relationship, but they can also cause boredom and monotony. Desire, by nature, thrives on the unusual and strange.

To keep desire alive, couples must intentionally interrupt their routines. This does not imply making major changes, but rather finding subtle ways to introduce freshness and excitement. This might be as easy as participating in a new hobby together, going on a spontaneous trip, or exploring new aspects of their sexuality. Couples can keep their relationship dynamic and their love for one other alive by constantly pursuing new experiences together.

The Dynamic Nature of Desire.
Desire is not a static force; it evolves and changes with time. What sparks passion in the beginning of a relationship may differ substantially from what keeps it going years later. Understanding this dynamic nature is essential for having a satisfying sexual connection.

Couples must be willing to explore new parts of their sexuality and adapt to changes in their wants. This could include having continuing discussions about their needs and desires, experimenting with new forms of intimacy, or finding external resources like therapy or workshops to help them better understand desire.

Embracing the paradox
The contradiction of love and desire is a fact that must be accepted rather than addressed. Couples can establish a more nuanced and meaningful relationship by identifying and respecting their diverse demands for closeness and passion. It necessitates a dedication to continuous effort, communication, and a willingness to accept the intricacies of human desire.

In the next chapters, we will explore deeper into the various aspects of this paradox, including practical tactics and insights for growing erotic intelligence and maintaining desire in long-term partnerships. Couples can learn how to maintain a spark of passion while fostering strong links of love and tenderness on this trip.

There is a natural contradiction between the ideals we seek in a long-term relationship — stability, trust, closeness — and the things that thrill us sexually — danger, unattainability, the strange, and unknown.

Love appreciates knowing everything about you, whereas desire requires mystery. Love tends to shorten the distance between me and you, whereas desire is fueled by it. Repetition numbs eroticism, yet familiarity and repetition foster intimacy. It lives on mystery, novelty, and the unexpected. Love is about having, whereas desire is about wanting. Desire, as an expression of longing, necessitates continued elusiveness. It is less concerned with where it has already been and more excited about where it can go.

When I initially read this, I thought, "Damn, that's an important thing to figure out." These two extremely crucial aspects of a relationship are in direct opposition with one another. On one side, we have a need for intimacy. A sense of knowing, trust, and certainty in the other. On the other hand, we have a longing for romance. A sense of intensity, mystery, and uncertainty.

Couples tend to go toward the closeness side of the spectrum rather than the desire side as time passes. People settle into their relationships. How often do you think you know everything there is to know about your spouse? What his thoughts are on this subject, and how she will react to that concept.
Furthermore, parenting advice frequently emphasizes the necessity of consistency and predictability for children. Parents need to be consistent and dependable. Not how you'd typically characterize a lover.

You can have both in a marriage.

Inertia forces us to pursue the path of least resistance, therefore it requires intention.

It takes skill to transition between the various roles required of us. The caregiver, event planner, confidant, breadwinner, and lover. A relationship isn't supposed to be everything at all times. We can adjust our relationship with our spouse to meet our needs and desires. Togetherness develops trust and affection. We also require sufficient distance to permit pursuit and mystery. They have distinct motivations and meet various requirements.

"Unbridled eroticism results in sex without attachment." In its most promiscuous and hedonistic form, it is unfulfilling and empty. Unbridled intimacy, on the other hand, fades into a dull gray. It's neat, safe, and unimaginative."

Individually, the search of intimacy and eroticism both result in disappointment. Intimacy and eroticism complement each other to form a constantly changing, dynamic relationship. Everything is just as God intended.

The Mystery of Erotic Intelligence

Erotic intelligence is a concept that includes far more than just sexual technique or frequency. It digs into the complex interplay between emotional connection and sexual desire, challenging us to discover the depths of our own and our partner's erotic identities. At its foundation, erotic intelligence is about understanding and fostering the ingredients that allow desire to grow, particularly in the setting of a committed relationship.

Understanding Erotic Intelligence

Erotic intelligence entails a profound understanding of the complexities and nuances of human desire. It is necessary to recognize that desire is a bodily, emotional, and psychological response. This intelligence focuses on:

Curiosity means taking an active interest in your partner's thoughts, feelings, and desires. Curiosity keeps the connection lively and avoids boredom.

Playfulness: Incorporating playfulness into the relationship helps reignite the spontaneity and excitement that are common in the early stages of romance.

Allowing oneself to be vulnerable is necessary for developing profound emotional and sexual closeness. It requires the courage to express your deepest thoughts and ambitions without fear of being judged.

Open, honest discussion about wants, dreams, and boundaries is essential. It fosters trust and helps partners manage the complexity of their sexual connection.

Imagination: The ability to imagine and fantasize is an important aspect of erotic intelligence. It helps people to explore their desires in a safe and creative setting.

The Role of Mystery in Desire

Erotic intelligence understands the paradoxical nature of desire: it often flourishes in the context of mystery and novelty. While love seeks to know and to be known, desire is drawn to what is unknown and elusive. This doesn't mean that partners need to hide secrets from each other, but rather that retaining a sense of individuality and personal space can improve desire.

Cultivating erotic intelligence

Developing erotic intelligence is a continuous process that involves both effort and intention. Practical steps for developing this intelligence include:

- ☐ Mindfulness: Practicing mindfulness can boost your awareness of your own desires and those of your spouse. It fosters being present in the moment and totally participating with your partner.
- ☐ Therapy and Education: Seeking tools such as books, workshops, or therapy can provide helpful insights into maintaining desire and handling sexual issues.
- ☐ Regular Check-ins: Regular chats about your relationship and sexual wants can help keep both parties aware of each other's needs and avoid misunderstandings.

Erotic intelligence's mystery rests in its ability to combine the familiar and the novel, the known and the unknown. It necessitates a complex knowledge of desire and a dedication to fostering it through inquiry, playfulness, vulnerability, and open communication. Couples can maintain a passionate and happy relationship throughout time by accepting the complexity of desire and striking a balance between intimacy and independence.

There is a strong propensity in long-term partnerships to favor the predictable over the surprising. Erotic passion is defiant and unexpected, unruly and undependable -- which leaves many people feeling separate and vulnerable. , "It is not true that romanticism fades with time. It gets riskier."

The irony is that regularity in even the most mundane marriages is an illusion. "Safety is presumed, not a given, but a construction." The belief that one's spouse is both safe and uninteresting is a creation that both parties have implicitly consented to and provides a false sense of security. People frequently engage in affairs in order to escape what they believe to be expected monotony. When the "dull partner" has an affair, the other is usually astonished. This is because the seemingly familiar spouse is actually enigmatic and unfamiliar.

It is commonly considered that intimacy and trust are required before sex can be enjoyed, yet for many men and, yes, even women, intimacy sabotages sexual desire. When a loved one is invested in the rewards of intimacy, such as security and stability, he or she may become desexualized, losing the urge to chase the fruits of passion.

Physical pleasure provides a unique shelter for many men and women; the body's soothing qualities allow for uninhibited expression. Only during sex can they get relief from their fears and compulsive ruminations. The physical pleasure drowns out the numbing worry of the day. It offers peace, self-revelation, and a sense of belonging.

Reconciliating Intimacy and Passion

The Initial Spark and its Evolution

The beginning of a relationship is frequently characterized by tremendous passion and desire. This initial spark is driven by novelty, mystery, and the thrill of discovery. However, as the relationship grows, the strength of this passion frequently decreases. While growing familiarity between couples deepens emotional connection, it can also reduce sexual desire. Reconciling intimacy and passion entails preserving the original spark while establishing a deep, persistent emotional connection.

The Nature of Intimacy

Intimacy is a profound emotional connection marked by trust, understanding, and mutual respect. It develops over time via shared experiences, open communication, and vulnerability. Intimacy lays the groundwork for a healthy and loving relationship, giving partners a safe area to express themselves and their needs.

Key elements of intimacy include:

- Emotional Support: Being present for one another at life's ups and downs, providing comfort, empathy, and understanding.
- Communication entails having honest and open discussions about feelings, opinions, and desires. Effective communication promotes trust and makes both partners feel heard and valued.

- Shared Experiences: Making memories together via common hobbies and interests. These events deepen the link between partners and promote a sense of unity.

The Nature of Passion.
In contrast, passion is motivated by desire, excitement, and novelty. It thrives on aspects of surprise, risk, and even a hint of danger. Passion is all about the thrill of the unknown and the joy of discovery. The main components of

Passion is introducing novel experiences and activities to keep relationships fresh and intriguing.
- Desire: Maintaining physical and emotional attraction to one another. This can be fostered through physical contact, flirting, and expressing sexual wants.
- Mystery: Maintaining a sense of uniqueness and unpredictability can increase desire. Allowing some room for personal development and freedom can provide a sense of intrigue.

Strategies for balancing intimacy and passion
Conciliating intimacy and desire entails striking a balance between these two critical components of a relationship. Here are some strategies to help you keep both.

Establish regular rituals that promote intimacy and connection. This might be a weekly date night, morning coffee together, or bedtime talks. These rituals allow opportunities to reconnect and develop your emotional attachment.

- Introduce Novelty: To keep the relationship active, introduce new experiences. Try new activities, visit new places, or experiment with new types of intimacy. Novelty can rekindle passion and keep the relationship fresh.
- Maintain Individuality: Encourage one another to pursue individual interests and personal development. Maintaining your sense of self can create a healthy distance that stimulates desire. When partners have separate passions and pursuits, they contribute new energy and perspectives to the partnership.
- Practice Vulnerability: Being open and vulnerable with one another promotes intimacy and trust. Express your worries, dreams, and desires openly. Vulnerability encourages a deeper emotional connection, which can lead to increased sexual closeness.
- Prioritize Physical Affection: Physical touch is an effective approach to maintain connection and arouse desire. Make an attempt to show regular physical affection, such as holding hands, embracing, kissing, or cuddling. Physical touch promotes connection and keeps the spark alive.
- Communicate About Sex: Talk openly and honestly about your sexual desires, boundaries, and dreams. Regular discussion regarding sex ensures that both partners feel fulfilled and understood. It also provides possibilities to explore new parts of your sexual connection.
- Balance Predictability and Spontaneity: Routines and predictability provide a sense of security, but

spontaneous moments can keep the relationship interesting. Surprise your partner with unexpected gestures, set up spontaneous dates, or try new activities together.

Reconciling intimacy and passion is a delicate balance that necessitates work, discussion, and a willingness to accept the intricacies of human desire. Couples can develop a meaningful and dynamic relationship by nurturing emotional connection as well as physical passion. The goal is to continually investing in both sides, maintaining the deep emotional connection while also igniting the spark of desire. Couples can experience a long-lasting, passionate partnership by navigating the natural ebbs and flows of desire with curiosity, fun, vulnerability, and open communication.

Let's be honest, the limerence phase is usually where our favorite rom-com flicks begin and end; we rarely see the loving pair transition onto the next chapter of their lives (and relationship).

We understand that in order for the relationship to continue, it must go to Phase 1: Building Trust and Phase 3: Building Commitment and Loyalty. It is entirely natural in long-term partnerships to seek components of the limerence period, particularly passion and intimacy. The wonderful thing is that we can renew the love and intimacy without the discomfort and preoccupation of the limerence phase (win-win!). Here are four strategies to reignite the romance in your relationship:

1. Practice emotional attunement.

Emotional attunement is the superpower of relationships! To attune to something is to become harmonious, conscious, or receptive to it. To be emotionally attuned means to be able to connect with our partner on a deeper level, or to enter someone's inner world. Attunement allows you to see the world from your partner's perspective and walk in their shoes. This allows you to sympathize with your spouse by listening to and observing their emotional cues, which fosters a stronger sense of connection.

Sometimes we say, "Get emotionally naked." That is, show and share your weaknesses with your spouse so that you can be really present with them in an emotional environment. Understanding your own emotions allows you to better understand and respond to those of your partner.

When we feel seen and understood, we feel closer, safer, and more deeply linked to our partner. Open-ended inquiries are an excellent approach to connect emotionally. That is, "if you offer questions that demand merely a yes or no answer, you are ruining conversations before they even have started. You accidently bang the door you are attempting to open.

2. Make intimacy a priority.

The older we become and the longer our relationship/marriage lasts, the more our thoughts and attention go to other aspects of our lives rather than each other. Whether it's worrying about finishing that work project, getting the kids to basketball practice, or catching up on our favorite Netflix show, romance and intimacy don't come as easily as they did when you first started dating and can often be the last thing on our "to do list" (if it even makes the list!). Have an open talk with your partner about methods to prioritize intimacy in your life, such as increasing date evenings, learning something new together, or establishing a rule of no TV in the bedroom after 9 p.m. Make intimacy a priority by modifying your routine and behaviors that are keeping you locked in ruts.

3. Increase the affectionate touch.

While sexual touch is crucial, non-sexual physical interaction appears to offer distinct advantages. Affectionate touch, such as holding hands or exchanging kisses, can occur on a daily basis and have incredible benefits for the health of your relationship. "Holding hands, hugging, and touching can release oxytocin, causing a calming sensation" - an excellent approach to relieve cortisol (a stress hormone) that has accumulated throughout a long and stressful work day.

As we go about our busy days, a kiss can quickly become a hello or goodbye. When we stop and lengthen the kiss (6 seconds or more), we allow ourselves to be present with our spouse and develop a stronger connection.

4. Date one another.

Too often, some people in a relationship hold the mistaken assumption that courtship and dating are reserved for the early years. When we are in the limerence phase, as seen in the aforementioned rom-coms, we date, flirt, and woo in an attempt to connect with one another. We somehow came to the conclusion that once we've done that, married, and had children, it's no longer necessary to date each other like we did in the beginning. Nothing could be farther from the truth. Setting aside sacred time (reference number 2) to pursue your mate is critical to long-term fulfillment in the relationship. Pro tip: Do something interesting or unusual together, and watch the sparks fly!

Here are some enjoyable date nights to take you out of your comfort zone:

Activities include paint-and-sip, laser tag, and dance/cooking workshops and Going to hear live music.

Chapter 2: The Myth of Spontaneous Sex

In popular culture, spontaneous sex is frequently portrayed as the ideal — a natural, easy expression of desire that occurs without prior planning or deliberation. This image implies that true desire is always spontaneous, and that sexual experiences should be fluid and unrestricted. However, this misconception can create undue expectations and pressure on couples, resulting in dissatisfaction and disappointment when real-life experiences fall short.

In reality, spontaneous sex is rarely as simple as it appears in films or television shows. Desire and arousal can take deliberate effort and development, particularly in long-term partnerships. Understanding this can help couples moderate their expectations and devise healthier, more realistic techniques to sustaining passion and intimacy.

Myths around spontaneity

Is spontaneous sex more satisfying? Although spontaneity may be a sign of passion for some, it can also have negative consequences. Although desire for sex can be great in the early stages of a new relationship, and sex may appear to occur spontaneously, sexual desire (and frequency of sex) frequently decreases over time in a partnership.

Long-term couples that wait for both partners to have a simultaneous rush of desire before having sex may rarely have intercourse.

Even if scheduling a sexual encounter is viewed as less seductive, planning may be required for sex to occur in the midst of other time constraints. Knowing when to have sex can also help people prepare for it — clothing, lubricant, seclusion — which may improve the experience.

Overcoming the Myth

To overcome the myth of spontaneous sex, couples must change their thinking and implement tactics that promote intentional connection. Here are a few practical approaches:

Communicate openly. Honest discussions about sexual needs, desires, and expectations are essential. This allows partners to better understand one other and coordinate their efforts to maintain a fulfilling sex life.

Plan intimacy. Planning intimate moments does not imply the loss of desire. On the contrary, anticipation can arouse desire and excitement. Couples can ensure that their sexual demands are addressed despite their hectic schedules by planning ahead of time.

Experiment together: Trying new activities together can renew the spirit of spontaneity and adventure. Experimentation, whether through novel sexual practices, role-playing, or the use of sex toys, can help to keep the relationship fresh and stimulating.

Create a relaxing environment. A suitable setting can improve intimacy. This could include creating a mood with lighting, music, or simply a clean and comfy bedroom. Creating a calm setting can make both lovers feel more connected and prepared for intimacy.

Prioritize self-care. Taking care of oneself physically and emotionally can boost sexual desire and performance. Exercise, proper food, and stress management can all lead to a happier and more fulfilling sexual life.

Maintain Physical Affection: Regular physical contact, such as embracing, kissing, and snuggling, can assist to maintain a connection and keep desire alive. These tiny acts of affection can lay the groundwork for more intimate encounters.

"In a new relationship, sex might feel effortless, but desire and frequency often decline over time."

spontaneity and satisfaction

In both studies, individuals believed that spontaneity was optimal. Contrary to popular assumption, spontaneous sex was not particularly satisfying.

In our first study, participants who were more closely associated with the spontaneity ideal reported being more sexually satisfied; nevertheless, when their most recent sexual experience was perceived to have occurred spontaneously, they found it no more satisfying than scheduled sex.

Planned sex can often be perceived as less sexy, but only by those who believe it is not ideal. Perceiving a recent sexual experience as planned was associated with poorer overall sexual pleasure, but this was not the case for those who strongly believed that planned sex was gratifying (yet, interestingly, one in every five said that their last sexual encounter was planned).

In a second study, we observed couples' sexual experiences over 21 days and found that sexual satisfaction was unaffected by whether sex was seen as spontaneous or planned, even among those who believed in the spontaneous sex ideal.

We also wanted to see how respondents felt spontaneity and planning affected their sexual experience. Interestingly, respondents said that spontaneity increased their sexual thrill, passion, purpose, and desire. However, several respondents said that preparing might increase anticipation and desire for sex.

And, while some people remarked that scheduled sex can add pressure, spontaneity is not necessarily the recipe for hot sex – some people claimed that when sex is unplanned, they may not have enough time to warm up to penetration, set aside mental distractions, or assure seclusion.

If sex is important to you and your partner(s), planning might help you prioritize your sexual connection. While the stars can sometimes align and create spur-of-the-moment desire, being purposeful about making time for sex can also pave the way for pleasant sexual encounters.

Planning sex does not need scheduling or sending out a calendar invite. It can be as simple as conversing with your partner to determine when the mood is most likely to occur, such as after sharing emotional intimacy or during less stressful hours at work, and agreeing to set aside time to connect.

With so many people still working from home or remotely, this might be as simple as adjusting your work hours to allow you to have an afternoon treat. In some situations, you or your spouse may choose to have sex in the morning or afternoon rather than at night, when you are ready to sleep after a large dinner.

Most couples use sex to maintain and deepen their relationship. And, like with date nights or weekend excursions, it may become necessary to plan in partnerships over time. The good news is that scheduled sex is just as likely to be enjoyable as spontaneous encounters.

The illusion of effortless desire

The Cultural Narrative

Popular culture frequently promotes the impression that sexual desire should be natural, uncomplicated, and constant. Movies, television shows, and novels regularly show couples having spontaneous, passionate sex with no apparent need for planning or effort. This cultural narrative implies that genuine love and desire should be spontaneous and automatic, requiring neither maintenance or conscious effort. However, this representation can be misleading and set unrealistic expectations for real-life relationships.

The Reality of Desire

Sexual desire is impacted by a wide range of internal and external influences. Stress, exhaustion, health concerns, emotional well-being, relationship dynamics, and life circumstances are all possible factors. Expecting desire to emerge naturally, without any nurturing or deliberate effort, is not only impractical, but can also lead to dissatisfaction and disappointment.

Factors Affecting Desire

High levels of stress and weariness can severely reduce sexual desire. Work stress, family duties, and day-to-day problems can all have an impact on one's sexual performance. Managing stress and getting enough rest are essential for having a strong sex drive.

- Health Issues: Physical health has a significant impact on sexual desire. Hormonal imbalances, chronic illnesses, and certain drugs can all have an effect on the libido. Maintaining excellent health through regular exercise, a balanced diet, and medical treatment is critical to sustaining desire.
- Emotional Well-Being: Emotional wellness is intimately related to sexual desire. Depression, worry, and low self-esteem can all make it difficult to feel sexually motivated. Addressing emotional difficulties with treatment, support, and self-care can help boost desire.
- Relationship Dynamics: The nature of the relationship might influence sexual desire. Conflicts, a lack of communication, and unresolved difficulties can lead to emotional distance and a decrease in desire. Building a

solid, trusting, and communicative relationship is critical to retaining passion.

The Effort Behind Desire

Sustaining sexual desire in a long-term relationship involves conscious effort and deliberate behaviors. Here are some basic tactics for sustaining and cultivating desire:

- ☐ Open communication is vital for discussing sexual needs, desires, and boundaries. Honest communication promotes understanding and enables partners to coordinate their efforts to meet each other's needs.
- ☐ Prioritizing closeness: Setting aside time for closeness is critical. This could include scheduling regular date nights, organizing romantic getaways, or simply making time for physical affection and connection.
- ☐ Creating A Conducive Environment: A relaxed and attractive setting might increase sexual desire. This could involve creating a relaxing atmosphere with music, soft lighting, and a distraction-free environment.
- ☐ Exploring New Experiences: Adding novelty and variation can help keep the relationship interesting. Trying new hobbies, experimenting with other forms of intimacy, or indulging in fantasies can rekindle passion.
- ☐ Maintaining Physical Affection: Physical touch, such as embracing, kissing, and snuggling, can help to keep a connection and desire alive. These tiny gestures of kindness increase intimacy and lay the groundwork for a stronger sexual connection.

☐ Investing in Emotional Intimacy: Creating a strong emotional link is essential for maintaining desire. This includes being present, demonstrating empathy, and supporting one another through life's obstacles.

Practical Steps for Couples

Couples can build and sustain desire by integrating effort into their daily lives.

Mindfulness practices can help you feel more present and connected in intimate moments. Meditation, deep breathing, and focusing on the present moment can increase awareness and enjoyment.

☐ Regular Check-ins: Having regular chats about the relationship and sexual needs can help both partners stay in sync with one other's desires. This can avoid misunderstandings and guarantee that both parties are satisfied.

☐ Physical and emotional self-care: Taking care of oneself is essential for sustaining desire. This encompasses both physical self-care (exercise and adequate nutrition) and emotional self-care (seeking treatment and engaging in enjoyable activities).

☐ Exploring Sensuality: Focusing on pleasurable activities other than sexual intercourse might enhance intimacy. Massages, showering together, and other sensory-based activities can help to foster connection.

Celebrating and appreciating small moments of connection and affection can serve as a foundation for deeper intimacy.

Recognizing and embracing these times strengthens the emotional bond and keeps the desire alive.

The appearance of effortless desire can lead to false expectations and unnecessary strain in relationships. Understanding that desire needs purposeful work and nurturing allows couples to establish healthier and more realistic approaches to maintaining closeness and passion. Embracing communication, emphasizing intimacy, and engaging in emotional connection are all effective tactics for maintaining desire over time. Recognizing the complexity of desire enables couples to develop a satisfying and dynamic sexual connection that evolves and deepens throughout time.

"Everyone seems to have it all figured out!" "Why can everyone do it but me?" Moving beyond perfectionism and resisting wellness performance. Breaking the illusion of uncomplicated desires.

In today's digital world, where we can all put our lives on show, the urge to broadcast and display particular elements of ourselves has become a recurring subject.

In a way, it's as if each of us is running our own cable news show, but we're the actor, director, and producer. There is a social pressure to present oneself in a positive light—the more intentional, desirable, and effortless your life appears to be, the more people want to listen in.

People are showcasing their picture-perfect healthy lifestyles on social media, from inspiring morning routines to mental health tips, and from "what-I-eat-in-a-day" videos to extremely clean houses. These people we encounter appear to have it all together, providing an appearance of effortless wellbeing that can make many of us feel inadequate, unable, and not good enough.

While I could write on how the wellness sector and health influencers are changing culture, that is not the focus of this essay. Recently, I've noticed how these tendencies are influencing the audience. While some people share their healthy habits online, the audience and viewers may feel compelled to live the same way others do.

Wellness and leading a healthy lifestyle are not as simple as the people you follow online make it appear. No one, including those who appear to have mastered wellness, has all the answers. Though they inspire us and show us what is possible, the people you see behind your screens are also human. They make mistakes. They have horrible days. They experience strong emotions. They also aim to interrupt negative cycles.

The self-imposed expectation to be like the individuals we see online may be keeping us trapped and holding us back. Hearing that other people online are human just like you are might feel unsettling at first, especially if you've grown to idolize or romanticize their life as compared to yours. In a way, it bursts our bubble, right? It breaks the illusion we've created in our minds of who we think they are. It reminds me of

Dorothy's reaction in the Wizard of Oz, when the curtain is pulled back to reveal the reality about "the magic" of Oz.

The Role of Routine and Novelty

The Balance Between Stability and Excitement.

Maintaining a balance between habit and novelty is essential for long-term connection and passion. Routine gives stability, security, and predictability, which are necessary for developing trust and emotional connection. Novelty, on the other hand, brings excitement, unpredictability, and a sense of adventure, which can rekindle passion and keep the relationship alive.

Routine can help build a solid and secure relationship, despite its perceived mundaneness. Here are some major advantages of routine:

- ☐ Building trust: Consistent habits and traditions help partners develop trust. Knowing what to expect from one another provides a stable and dependable basis for the partnership.
- ☐ Creating Connection: Regular routines, such as shared meals, nightly walks, and nighttime rituals, provide for connection and communication. These moments of closeness deepen the emotional connection.
- ☐ Predictable routines can help to alleviate stress and promote a sense of order and serenity in daily life. This consistency makes partners feel more at ease and focused on developing their relationship.
- ☐ Establishing rituals displays dedication to the partnership. It demonstrates that both couples are invested in preserving and growing their relationship.

The Power of Novelty

While routine is vital, bringing innovation is also necessary to keep the relationship interesting and passionate. Here's how novelty may enhance a relationship:

- ☐ Enhancing enthusiasm: New experiences and activities can rekindle the enthusiasm and passion that are common in the early stages of a relationship. Novelty increases dopamine production, which is linked to pleasure and reward.
- ☐ Preventing Boredom: Trying new and different activities keeps the relationship from becoming static. Novelty keeps the relationship interesting and avoids boredom from settling in.
- ☐ Encouraging Growth: Trying new things together promotes personal and interpersonal development. It enables partners to learn more about one another and uncover new elements of their personalities and interests.
- ☐ Sharing unique experiences creates enduring memories and stories that partners may reminisce over, which strengthens their bond even more.

Strategies for Integrating Routine and Novelty

To successfully integrate regularity and novelty, you must be intentional and willing to explore and adapt. Here are some techniques for keeping the balance:

Establish regular rituals that promote connection and closeness. This may be a weekly date night, a daily check-in, or a monthly outing together. These rituals promote stability while also allowing for connection.

- ☐ Plan for Spontaneity: Although it may appear contradictory, preparing for spontaneity entails deliberately providing possibilities for spontaneous actions. This could include making time for spontaneous adventures or compiling a list of exciting activities to attempt together.

- ☐ Change up routines: Make tiny alterations to your regular routine to keep things interesting. This could include attempting a new supper recipe, going a different route on your usual stroll, or changing up your workout program.

- ☐ Pursue New Interests Together: Try new hobbies or activities as a couple. This could be attending a dance class, learning a new language, or traveling to new places. Shared interests generate enthusiasm and offer new possibilities to interact.

- ☐ Surprise Each Other: Create surprises for each other to keep the relationship interesting. These surprises don't have to be large gestures; even tiny, thoughtful deeds can add to the thrill and demonstrate that you care about one another.

- ☐ Maintain Individuality: Encourage one another to pursue individual interests and personal development. Separate activities and experiences bring new energy and views into the partnership, increasing intimacy and desire.

Practical Examples of Routine and Novelty

- Routine: A couple may build a habit of eating breakfast together every morning. This time can be utilized to connect, discuss the day's goals, and express any relevant thoughts or sentiments. This practice offers a continuous opportunity to connect.
- Novelty: To provide variety, the same pair may opt to try a new sort of cuisine once a month. This may include preparing a new cuisine at home or visiting a restaurant they've never been to before. This shared experience generates enthusiasm and fresh memories.
- Routine: Establishing a nighttime ritual, such as reading a book together or sharing a moment of appreciation before going to bed, can foster feelings of connection and security.
- Novelty: Taking a spontaneous weekend excursion to a nearby city or countryside might relieve the monotony and provide an opportunity for exploration and bonding.

Overcoming Challenges

Balancing habit with novelty can be difficult, particularly in the face of hectic schedules, stress, and life upheavals. Here are some suggestions for solving these challenges:

Communicate openly. Discuss the value of both routine and novelty with your partner. Share your needs and desires, and then listen to your partner's perspective. Open communication guarantees that both partners are on the same page and dedicated to keeping the balance.

Be flexible: Life is unpredictable, thus adaptability is essential. Be open to change and tweak your habits and plans as necessary. Flexibility enables you to adapt to changes without becoming overwhelmed or stressed.

Prioritize Quality Time: Prioritize quality time together, even if it means scheduling it on your schedule. Protecting this time from other responsibilities demonstrates how vital your relationship is.

Celebrate small wins: Recognize and applaud the modest steps you both do to maintain routine and introduce novelty. These celebrations reinforce healthy behaviors and express gratitude for one another's efforts.

Seek Help: If balancing regularity and novelty becomes challenging, try consulting a therapist or counselor. Professional advice can offer new perspectives and ideas for keeping a healthy and vibrant relationship.

In long-term partnerships, maintaining closeness and desire requires a mix of habit and novelty. Routine gives the stability and security necessary to foster trust and emotional connection, whereas novelty adds excitement and keeps the relationship dynamic. Couples can actively integrate these qualities to create a rich and fulfilling relationship that changes and grows over time. Partners may negotiate the complications of maintaining routine and novelty by communicating openly, being flexible, and committing to each other's well-being. This ensures an enduring and passionate relationship.

Boredom in old age can be a dangerous and destructive thing, and, while we do not advocate abandoning the safe and familiar, discovering what novelty truly means may help to enrich people's experiences in their golden years; we hope that the work we are doing will help to bring this to light.

Chapter 3: From Adventure to Ambivalence

In the early phases of a relationship, the sense of adventure and discovery is typically thrilling. New experiences, shared firsts, and the joy of learning about one another foster a deep bond powered by enthusiasm and curiosity. This moment, also known as the "honeymoon phase," is marked by powerful emotions and a strong sense of connection.

However, as partnerships grow, the initial enthusiasm fades into routine, and partners may become uncertain about their connection. The change from adventure to ambivalence is a normal phase of relationship development, but it can be difficult to negotiate.

The honeymoon phase

The honeymoon phase is characterized by:

- Intense Attraction: Physical and emotional attraction are at their pinnacle. Couples typically feel strongly attached and have a great desire to be together.
- Novelty and exploration: Everything feels fresh and intriguing. Couples enjoy discovering one another's interests, preferences, and personalities.
- Idealization: Partners often see each other in an idealized perspective, emphasizing positive attributes and ignoring shortcomings.
- High Levels of Intimacy: Emotional and physical intimacy are strong, with frequent displays of love and affection.

The onset of ambiguity

As the relationship evolves, various variables can lead to the emergence of ambivalence:

- ☐ Familiarity and Routine: As partners become more comfortable with one another, the sensation of novelty fades. Routine and predictability have replaced the exhilaration of fresh encounters.
- ☐ Flaws Emerge: As time passes, spouses become more conscious of one another's flaws and shortcomings. The idyllic image fades as reality settles in.
- ☐ External stressors: Work, family commitments, and financial worries can all have an affect on the relationship. These circumstances can limit the time and energy available to maintain intimacy.
- ☐ Emotional Distance: As the initial passion fades, emotional distance may emerge. Partners may feel less connected and more focused on their respective goals.

Understanding Ambivalence

Ambivalence in relationships is a state of conflicting emotions and uncertainty. It involves conflicting emotions, since partners may have both positive and bad feelings toward each other and the relationship. Understanding ambivalence is essential for navigating this difficult phase.

- ☐ Normalizing Ambivalence: Understanding that ambivalence is a natural element of long-term partnerships can help to alleviate feelings of fear and inadequacy. It is normal for feelings to fluctuate over time.

- ☐ Identifying Underlying Causes: Reflecting on the elements that contribute to ambivalence might help you understand the relationship. Understanding the causes is the first step toward resolving them.
- ☐ Open Communication: Discussing ambivalence with a spouse might help you understand and empathize. Open communication enables partners to manage this phase jointly.

Strategies for Rekindling Adventure.

Rekindling a spirit of adventure in a relationship might help you overcome ambivalence and regain closeness and connection. Here are some ways to rekindle passion and excitement:

Introduce novelty. Actively look for new experiences and activities to share. This could include visiting new areas, trying new activities, or pursuing new interests together.

Prioritize quality time. Set aside time for each other, free of distractions. Prioritizing quality time can deepen emotional bonds and provide possibilities for connection.

Create shared goals. Setting common goals and working toward them can foster a sense of collaboration and purpose. Working together builds connection, whether it's to plan a future vacation, begin a project, or set personal goals.

Express Appreciation: Regularly expressing appreciation and gratitude to one another strengthens positive thoughts and counteracts negative. Small expressions of gratitude can have a tremendous impact on the relationship.

Engage in physical affection. Physical touch is an effective approach to sustain intimacy. Regular physical affection, such as hugging, kissing, and snuggling, can help to deepen the emotional bond.

Relationships can be difficult, but with patience, perseverance, and open communication, you can develop a happier and more rewarding connection. Remember that you deserve to be loved and respected, and your decisions should always reflect what is best for you and your well-being.

When to Break It Off.
While each sort of relationship presents its unique set of issues, here are some signals that it may be time to end your relationship:

You don't feel anything change. Your doubts and concerns linger, and little progress has been achieved despite open conversation and competent assistance.

Talking with your lover is like pulling teeth. Your apathetic partner refuses to accept and address your worries.

You are usually stressed. The connection consistently causes you to feel stressed, anxious, or depressed.

Your lives are heading in several directions: You have incompatible aims, values, or lifestyles.

Love is no longer part of the relationship. You no longer feel supported or loved in this relationship.

You feel taken for granted: your needs aren't being addressed, and your spouse doesn't appreciate the effort you put into the relationship. You feel like you're doing all the heavy work, which may lower your self-esteem.

You no longer have common interests. Your relationship is becoming more strained, and there are fewer and fewer things that make you happy together.

Your gut suggests you should leave: When it's time for a change, your body usually knows first. If something doesn't feel right, follow your instincts and look for signals that it's time to move on.

You no longer trust each other. When communication becomes less open and honest, trust in a relationship can swiftly deteriorate.

Breaking up is never an easy decision, but remember that you deserve to be in a healthy, satisfying relationship. Trust your intuition and prioritize your health. Remember that with time and self-care, you can heal and move on to a better, healthier future with the right partner.

How To End A Relationship

If, after reading this article, you believe it is time to terminate your love relationship, here are some suggestions to assist make the process as painless as possible:

Be honest and direct. When terminating a relationship, it is critical to explain your feelings honestly and completely to your partner. While it may be tough, phrasing the conversation in a respectful and understanding manner can make both parties feel heard.

Take care of yourself. Ending a relationship can be emotionally demanding, so make time for yourself and practice self-care. During this transition period, make an effort to engage in activities that will assist you in dealing with your emotions and recharge.

Keep busy: Don't waste time at home; instead, spend it doing something you enjoy. Take part in events with your friends and family, or volunteer with a local charity. Keeping occupied might help to alleviate feelings of loneliness and boredom.

Allow yourself to grieve: It is critical to take the time necessary to process the emotions associated with the termination of a relationship. Allow yourself to be upset and furious, but also realize that you are resilient and capable of moving forward.

Seek professional help: Speaking with a therapist or counselor can be quite beneficial during the transition time after ending a relationship. They can offer support, counsel, and perspective when dealing with the emotions that come with terminating a relationship.

Be gentle to yourself: Above all, remember that you are doing your best for yourself and your future. Stay cheerful and look forward to brighter times!

Discover Your and Your Partner's Attachment Style.

Several attachment theories describe how early childhood experiences influence adult love relationships. Understanding your attachment style and that of your partner (and other close relationships!) allows you to better spot actions that lead to unhealthy relationship patterns. This understanding can then be applied to promote growth and good transformation in areas such as communication, trust, and emotional connection.

Final Thoughts

Managing ambivalence in a relationship can be difficult and unpredictable. Emotions are strong, and you're probably puzzled about whether you should persevere or give up.

Breaking up a relationship can be difficult and traumatic, but with the correct care and support, you can move on. To protect your emotional well-being during this period, seek expert help and allow yourself to process challenging emotions.

Navigating the Journey from Courtship to Commitment

The excitement of courtship

Courtship is generally the most exciting part of a romantic relationship. It has the following characteristics:

Passion and infatuation: During romance, emotions are intense. Partners are passionately enamored, with strong attraction and passion. The exhilaration of new love drives this period, making everything feel lively and urgent.

Courtship is about investigating and finding each other's personalities, likes, dislikes, and life stories. Each new piece of information feels like a treasure, adding to the sensation of discovery and adventure.

Idealization: Partners frequently see each other through rose-colored glasses, focusing on favorable characteristics while downplaying or disregarding problems. This idealization aids in establishing a strong initial bond.

Frequent Interaction: During courtship, partners typically spend a lot of time together, participating in numerous activities, going on dates, and chatting regularly to strengthen their bond.

The Transition to Commitment.

As the relationship advances from courting to commitment, various changes and challenges occur:

Commitment necessitates a deeper emotional relationship than first interest. This entails understanding each other's needs, supporting each other's objectives, and sharing weaknesses.

Facing Reality: Idealization fades when partners come to see each other more realistically. This phase entails accepting one another's shortcomings and imperfections.

Building Trust: Trust becomes an essential component of committed relationships. This includes being trustworthy, honest, and showing integrity in both acts and words.

Navigating Conflicts: Conflict is unavoidable in any relationship. Learning how to negotiate disagreements and settle conflicts constructively is critical for long-term commitment.

Key Components of Commitment

- ☐ Mutual Respect: Respect for one other's uniqueness, opinions, and boundaries is essential. This regard promotes a healthy, balanced partnership.
- ☐ Shared Values and Goals: Having matched values and goals promotes the relationship. Partners should talk about and agree on important parts of life, such as family, profession, income, and lifestyle.
- ☐ Effective Communication: Open, honest, and compassionate communication is essential for a lasting

connection. This includes actively listening, expressing views and feelings clearly, and being open to feedback.

- ☐ Emotional connection: Deep emotional connection extends beyond physical attractiveness. Sharing worries, dreams, and experiences fosters a close emotional tie.
- ☐ Support and Encouragement: Fostering one other's personal development and enjoying victories together lays the groundwork for encouragement and partnership.

Strategies to Strengthen Commitment

- ☐ Cultivating trust requires continuous and reliable activities. Keeping promises, being truthful, and demonstrating dependability build trust.
- ☐ Prioritize Quality Time: Spending quality time together creates emotional bonds. This can include regular date nights, similar interests, and meaningful talks.
- ☐ Practice Forgiveness: Mistakes and misunderstandings occur. Forgiveness and letting go of grudges are critical to maintaining a successful relationship.
- ☐ Show Appreciation: Regularly expressing appreciation and thanks promotes positivity. Small acts of kindness and acknowledgment go a long way towards establishing commitment.
- ☐ Maintain Physical Intimacy: Physical closeness, including affection and sexual intimacy, is essential for a lasting partnership. It strengthens the emotional connection and keeps the passion alive.

Navigating the path from courting to commitment entails moving from the thrill of new love to the formation of a stable, permanent partnership. This process necessitates strengthening emotional bonds, establishing trust, and learning how to resolve disagreements constructively. Couples can improve their commitment and develop a successful, long-term relationship by establishing mutual respect, good communication, emotional intimacy, and support. While obstacles are unavoidable, approaching them with empathy, flexibility, and a willingness to seek assistance when necessary may keep the connection strong and durable. The rewards of commitment, such as deeper love, emotional security, shared life experiences, and personal growth, make the journey worthwhile, resulting in a long-lasting connection.

Marriage is a lovely and rewarding experience, but it also presents its own set of problems. Whether you are freshly married or thinking about getting married, understanding the distinctions between single and married life is critical.

Traditionally, it entails getting to know one other, spending time together, and discovering each other's values and beliefs. As the relationship evolves, the pair may start dating and eventually become engaged.

Getting married is a pivotal milestone in anyone's life. It represents a big commitment to someone you love and intend to spend the rest of your life with.

Being married differs from being single, in which you just have yourself to care for. When you're married, you have someone else to consult with and agree on things that affect both of your lives, such as finances, health, and important life choices.

Loyalty, time commitment, gift-giving, and romantic activities are among the commonalities between serious dating and marriage. Just because you are married does not imply your courtship is over.

Spending quality time together, providing meaningful presents, and finding ways to surprise your mate with romantic gestures are all important steps toward a happy marriage.

Adjustments to a married lifestyle
Married life necessitates some adaptations. At its core, marriage is about creating a life together, which requires making sacrifices and concessions along the way.

Here are some of the changes you might need to make.
- ☐ Financial changes: When you marry, you will need to merge your finances and collaborate to make key decisions about spending, saving, and investing. This could include granting each other permission to make significant purchases or budgeting for shared spending.
- ☐ Changing priorities: Marriage requires you to construct a life together, which may entail giving up specific hobbies or interests to make room for shared ones. Communication and decision-making with partners: Being married requires you to discuss major decisions with your partner and ensure that your choices are consistent with your shared goals and values.
- ☐ Trust and openness in relationships: A trustworthy and healthy marriage should have no grey areas or secrets. This includes checking in with each other on a regular

basis, being honest about your feelings, and taking precautions to avoid infidelity.

☐ Embracing a married identity: Finally, you must embrace your married identity by wearing a wedding ring, utilizing married titles, and updating your marital status on vital documents.

To summarize, knowing the distinctions between single and married life, adjusting to a married lifestyle, planning for the future as a couple, and remaining loyal to your marriage vows are all critical components of a good and fulfilling marriage. You can live a life filled with joy, happiness, and shared experiences if you actively work to build a solid, supportive, and loving relationship with your significant other.

The path may have ups and downs, but if you remain committed to your relationship, you can effectively navigate it with your spouse by your side. Remember, a marriage is a collaboration, and it takes effort and attention to make it work, but the rewards are immense.

Chapter 4: The Pitfalls of Modern Romance

Modern romance is influenced by a multitude of factors that make it complex and often challenging. While technological advancements and changing social norms have opened up new avenues for connection, they have also introduced new pitfalls.

The Influence of Technology

- Online Dating: The rise of online dating platforms has transformed how people meet and form relationships. While these platforms increase opportunities to meet potential partners, they also present challenges:
- Overwhelm of Choice: An abundance of options can lead to decision paralysis and a tendency to view potential partners as disposable.
- Superficial Connections: Online profiles often emphasize physical appearance and brief bios, which can lead to shallow connections based on first impressions rather than deeper compatibility.
- Misrepresentation: The anonymity of online platforms can encourage misrepresentation, leading to mismatched expectations and disappointment.
- Digital Communication: Technology has made communication easier, but it has also introduced new challenges:
- Miscommunication: Text messages and social media interactions can lead to misunderstandings due to the lack of non-verbal cues.
- Constant Connectivity: The expectation of constant availability can create pressure and reduce personal space.

- Distracted Presence: The prevalence of smartphones and social media can result in partners being physically present but mentally distracted, leading to reduced quality of interactions.

Emotional and Psychological Challenges
- High Expectations: Modern romance is often burdened by unrealistic expectations:
- Idealized Love: Media and popular culture portray idealized versions of love and relationships, creating unrealistic standards that real-life relationships struggle to meet.
- Instant Gratification: The culture of instant gratification can lead to impatience and a lack of willingness to work through challenges in a relationship.
- Emotional Vulnerability: Navigating emotional vulnerability is a significant challenge:
- Fear of Rejection: Fear of rejection can hinder openness and honesty, leading to superficial interactions.
- Emotional Baggage: Past experiences and unresolved issues can impact current relationships, making it difficult to fully trust and commit.

Strategies for Navigating Modern Romance
- Effective Communication: Prioritizing clear, open, and empathetic communication is crucial. This includes discussing expectations, resolving conflicts, and expressing needs and feelings.
- Setting Boundaries: Establishing and respecting personal boundaries helps maintain individuality and

personal space within the relationship. This includes managing technology use and ensuring quality time together.

- Realistic Expectations: Developing realistic expectations based on mutual understanding rather than idealized notions of romance can reduce disappointment and increase satisfaction.
- Embracing Vulnerability: Being open and vulnerable with each other fosters deeper connections. This involves sharing fears, dreams, and insecurities and building trust over time.
- Balancing Individual and Relationship Goals: Finding a balance between personal growth and relationship goals ensures that both partners feel fulfilled and supported. This includes supporting each other's careers, hobbies, and personal aspirations.
- Navigating Cultural Differences: Approaching cultural differences with curiosity and respect can enrich the relationship. Open discussions about traditions, values, and expectations help in finding common ground.
- Managing Social Media Influence: Limiting the impact of social media on the relationship by focusing on real-life interactions and avoiding comparisons can improve relationship satisfaction.

The pitfalls of modern romance are multifaceted, influenced by technology, changing social norms, and evolving emotional and psychological dynamics. Navigating these challenges requires intentional effort, effective communication, and a willingness to embrace vulnerability and growth. By setting realistic expectations, balancing individual and relationship goals, and managing the influence of technology and social media, couples can build strong, fulfilling relationships in the contemporary world. Understanding and addressing these pitfalls can lead to deeper connections, increased satisfaction, and lasting love amidst the complexities of modern life.

The explosion of online dating apps has made meeting new people radically convenient. But more of those looking for love complain that the platforms take the romance out of dating and turn it into nothing but a game of odds. Perhaps that's why dating apps are losing their appeal, especially among Gen Z. According to one study, Gen Z-ers make up only 26% of dating app users. We'll discuss how different generations find connections and why it still might be possible to find romance online. What's been your experience with dating apps?

Balancing Independence and Togetherness
The art of maintaining a healthy and fulfilling relationship lies in finding the delicate equilibrium between two seemingly opposing forces: independence and togetherness. In this exploration, we delve into the intricate dynamics of relationships, dissecting the importance of both independence and togetherness, the challenges they can present, and strategies for achieving the perfect balance that nurtures love and personal growth.

The Yin and Yang of Relationships

- Independence: This represents the individual's need for autonomy, personal space, and self-expression. It's the desire to pursue personal interests, hobbies, and goals outside the relationship.
- Togetherness: On the other end of the spectrum, togetherness signifies the desire for closeness, intimacy, and shared experiences. It involves spending quality time together, making joint decisions, and building a life as a unit.

The Significance of Independence

Independence within a relationship is not a sign of detachment or a lack of commitment. Instead, it plays a pivotal role in the health and longevity of the partnership:

- Personal Growth: Independence allows individuals to continue growing, learning, and evolving. It ensures that personal goals and aspirations remain a driving force.
- Self-Identity: Maintaining one's individuality within a relationship is vital. It ensures that both partners retain a strong sense of self, which can enrich the relationship.
- Reducing Codependency: Overdependence on a partner can lead to codependency, which can be detrimental to the relationship. Independence helps mitigate this risk.
- Respecting Boundaries: Independence respects personal boundaries and acknowledges that each person has their own needs and desires.

The Importance of Togetherness

While independence is crucial, so is the need for togetherness:

☐ Building Bonds: Togetherness creates the foundation for intimacy and deep emotional connections. It's the glue that binds partners together through shared experiences.

☐ Teamwork: In a healthy relationship, couples work together as a team. Togetherness is essential for making joint decisions, tackling challenges, and achieving shared goals. One aspect that should not be ignored is increasing your daily habits and creating habits to reach goals. This is oA variety of factors influence modern romance, making it complex and often difficult to navigate. While technological advancements and shifting social norms have provided new opportunities for connection, they have also introduced new risks.

The Influence of Technology

☐ Online Dating: The proliferation of online dating sites has changed the way people meet and form relationships. While these platforms provide more opportunities to meet potential partners, they also pose challenges:

☐ Overwhelm of Choice: Too many possibilities can cause decision paralysis and a tendency to dismiss potential mates as disposable.

☐ Superficial interactions: Online profiles frequently stress physical attractiveness and brief bios, which can result in superficial interactions based on immediate impressions rather than deeper compatibility.

- ☐ Misrepresentation: The anonymity of internet platforms can foster misrepresentation, resulting in misaligned expectations and disillusionment.
- ☐ Digital Communication: Technology has simplified communication, but it has also presented new challenges:
- ☐ Miscommunication: The absence of nonverbal indicators in text messages and social media conversations can lead to misconceptions.
- ☐ Constant Connectivity: Expecting to be available at all times can put strain on one's personal space.
- ☐ preoccupied Presence: With the popularity of cellphones and social media, partners may be physically present but mentally preoccupied, resulting in lower-quality interactions.

Emotional and Psychological Challenges

- ☐ High Expectations: Modern romance is frequently saddled with false expectations.
- ☐ Idealized Love: Media and popular culture present idealized portrayals of love and relationships, resulting in false expectations that real-life partnerships fail to match.
- ☐ quick satisfaction: The culture of quick satisfaction can lead to frustration and a lack of motivation to work through issues in a relationship.
- ☐ Emotional Vulnerability: Navigating emotional fragility is a huge challenge:

- ☐ Fear of Rejection: Fear of rejection can hamper openness and honesty, resulting to shallow encounters.
- ☐ Emotional Baggage: Past experiences and unsolved difficulties can damage current relationships, making it harder to fully trust and commit.

Strategies for Navigating Modern Romance

- ☐ Effective communication requires a focus on clarity, openness, and empathy. This includes discussing expectations, resolving conflicts, and communicating needs and emotions.
- ☐ Setting Boundaries: Having and respecting personal boundaries helps to maintain individuality and personal space in a relationship. This includes managing technology usage and spending quality time together.
- ☐ Realistic Expectations: Developing realistic expectations based on mutual understanding, rather than idealized romantic notions, can reduce disappointment while increasing satisfaction.
- ☐ Embracing vulnerability: Being open and vulnerable with one another promotes deeper connections. This entails discussing one's concerns, dreams, and uncertainties while gradually gaining trust.
- ☐ Balance Individual and Relationship Goals: Achieving a balance between personal development and relationship goals guarantees that both parties are satisfied and supported. This involves supporting one another's careers, interests, and personal goals.
- ☐ Navigating Cultural Differences: Treating cultural differences with curiosity and respect can improve the

relationship. Open discussions about traditions, values, and expectations can help people find common ground.
- ☐ Managing Social Media Influence: By focusing on real-life interactions rather than comparisons, you can improve relationship satisfaction.

The pitfalls of modern romance are multifaceted, influenced by technology, changing social norms, and shifting emotional and psychological dynamics. Navigating these obstacles needs deliberate effort, excellent communication, and a willingness to accept vulnerability and growth. Couples can develop robust, meaningful relationships in today's environment by setting realistic expectations, balancing individual and relationship goals, and controlling the impact of technology and social media. Understanding and addressing these pitfalls can lead to deeper connections, increased satisfaction, and lasting love amidst the complexities of modern life.

The explosion of online dating apps has made meeting new people radically convenient. But more of those looking for love complain that the platforms take the romance out of dating and turn it into nothing but a game of odds. Perhaps that's why dating apps are losing their appeal, especially among Gen Z. According to one study, Gen Z-ers make up only 26% of dating app users. We'll address how various generations discover connections and why it still could be feasible to find romance online. What's been your experience using dating apps?

Balancing Independence and Togetherness

The art of maintaining a healthy and rewarding relationship involves striking a precise balance between two seemingly conflicting forces: independence and connection. In this exploration, we will look at the intricate dynamics of relationships, including the importance of independence and togetherness, the challenges they can present, and strategies for striking the perfect balance that fosters love and personal growth.

The yin and yang of relationships

- ☐ Independence symbolizes the individual's desire for autonomy, personal space, and self-expression. It is a desire to pursue personal interests, hobbies, and goals outside of the relationship.
- ☐ Togetherness: On the other end of the scale, togetherness symbolizes the desire for connection, intimacy, and shared experiences. It means spending quality time together, making joint decisions, and developing a life as a unit.

The Significance of Independence

- ☐ Independence within a relationship is not a sign of detachment or a lack of commitment. Instead, it plays a key role in the health and durability of the partnership:
- ☐ Personal Growth: Independence permits individuals to continue growing, learning, and evolving. It ensures that personal objectives and aspirations remain a motivating factor.

- ☐ Self-Identity: Maintaining one's individuality within a relationship is vital. It ensures that both partners maintain a strong sense of self, which can improve their relationship.
- ☐ Reducing Codependency: Overreliance on a partner can lead to codependency, which is harmful to the relationship. Independence helps to reduce this risk.
- ☐ Respecting Boundaries: Independence respects personal boundaries and recognizes that each individual has unique needs and desires.

- ☐ This might be a few minutes in the morning or evening to discuss thoughts, feelings, and reflections.
- ☐ Weekly Date Nights: Regular date evenings, even if they are modest and at home, might assist to keep the romance and novelty alive. Cooking a meal together, watching a movie, or participating in a common pastime can all help to maintain the connection.

Physical Touch and Affection

Maintaining physical touch and compassion in daily life is critical for sustaining passion.

- Non-Sexual Affection: Physical contact that is not sexual in nature, such as holding hands, embracing, or cuddling, promotes intimacy and connection. These affectionate actions serve as a reminder of their physical and emotional link.
- Allowing for spontaneous moments of intimacy, rather than waiting for the "right time," might help to maintain

the intensity. This could be a short kiss, a playful touch, or an unexpected embrace.

-

Prioritizing intimacy.

Maintaining desire requires prioritizing intimacy, especially in the middle of busy schedules and daily responsibilities:

- Scheduled Intimacy: While spontaneity is vital, setting aside time for intimacy can help to keep it a priority. This could include scheduling certain periods for physical intimacy or romantic activities.
- Emotional intimacy: Prioritizing emotional closeness by sharing your thoughts, dreams, and vulnerabilities strengthens your bond. Open and honest discussion about feelings and desires promotes intimacy and understanding.

Exploring Creativity Together

Incorporating creativity into daily life can revitalize a relationship and turn mundane activities into opportunities for connection and enjoyment:

- Creative Projects: Working on creative tasks together, such as painting, gardening, or home remodeling, can promote cooperation and a sense of accomplishment. These projects provide couples the opportunity to express themselves and create something special together.
- Cooking and experimenting in the kitchen: Trying new recipes or cooking techniques can make meal preparation a fun and social activity. Cooking together

promotes teamwork and provides an opportunity to experiment and have fun.

Shared goals and aspirations

Aligning on similar goals and working towards them together can foster a strong sense of togetherness and purpose.

- Fitness and health: Couples who commit to a fitness routine or health goal can benefit from mutual support and inspiration. Whether it's going to the gym, hiking, or practicing yoga, sharing physical activities can benefit both the body and the relationship.
- Financial Planning: Collaborating on financial objectives, such as saving for a vacation or budgeting for the future, can help couples keep on track and motivated. Open discussions about economics can alleviate stress and foster a sense of collaboration.

Celebrate Everyday Moments

Recognizing and praising little, everyday occurrences can help couples recognize the beauty in the ordinary:

- Morning and evening rituals: Creating small rituals, such as sharing a morning coffee or relaxing together in the evening, can help to foster important everyday ties. These routines allow us to start and conclude the day with love and appreciation.
- Acknowledging achievements: Celebrating one another's accomplishments, no matter how minor, develops an environment of support and pride. Recognizing and

applauding your partner's efforts and triumphs builds mutual respect and admiration.

The Power of Playfulness.

Revitalizing Relationships

Playfulness is an effective strategy for revitalizing relationships and instilling a feeling of adventure in everyday life. It creates a lighthearted mood that can reduce stress, boost connection, and increase intimacy. Here are some ways playfulness may improve relationships:

Engaging in entertaining activities helps to break up the monotony of daily tasks. Playfulness instills spontaneity and excitement in the relationship, keeping it dynamic and engaging. Simple gestures such as unexpected dance parties in the living room or humorous pillow fights can shake up the routine and inject new vitality into the relationship.

Reducing Stress: Playfulness can be a great stress reliever. Endorphins, which are natural mood boosters, are released when people laugh or interact playfully. When couples engage in playful activities, they develop a buffer against the stressors of everyday life, helping them to face obstacles with a lighter, more cheerful attitude.

Enhancing Communication

Playfulness can also improve communication in a partnership, making conversations more relaxed and open.

- Fostering Open Dialogue: Playful banter and humor can help to foster an environment conducive to open communication. When partners engage in fun talks, they are more likely to feel comfortable expressing themselves and addressing delicate themes. This ease of communicating can improve the emotional bond between spouses.

- Defusing Tension: Humor and playfulness can help to relieve tension during a fight. A well-timed joke or lighthearted gesture can lighten the mood and divert attention away from the conflict, making it easier to reconcile differences. Even during difficult times, playfulness can act as a reminder that the partnership can bring joy and friendship.

Building Emotional Intimacy

Playfulness promotes emotional intimacy by allowing couples to be themselves and enjoy each other's company:

- Creating shared memories: Playing together promotes great, shared memories. These encounters form part of the relationship's narrative, strengthening the bond between the couples. Whether it's trying new hobbies, traveling, or simply playing games, these moments of happiness and laughter enhance the bond.

- Encouraging vulnerability: Playfulness encourages partners to down their guard and be vulnerable with one another. When partners engage in playful relationships, they frequently let rid of self-consciousness and accept their true selves. This transparency promotes greater emotional intimacy and trust.

Stimulating physical intimacy.

Playfulness can also improve physical intimacy, resulting in a more comfortable and enjoyable environment for closeness.

Playful touches and gestures can start physical attachment in a non-threatening way. Tickling, playful wrestling, or simply holding hands while joking about can open the door to more personal interactions, making physical proximity feel normal and spontaneous.

Maintaining passion: Keeping the aspect of fun alive helps to preserve passion in the relationship. Playfulness can instill a sense of surprise and pleasure in physical closeness, keeping it from becoming ordinary or predictable. Trying new things together, joking at intimate moments, and not taking oneself too seriously can all help keep the desire alive.

Strengthening the bond with shared laughter

Shared laughing is one of the most deep manifestations of playfulness, and it plays an important role in developing the link between partners.

Creating inside jokes: Inside jokes are a unique and effective method to build intimacy. They create a secret world that only the partners comprehend, increasing feelings of belonging and connection. These shared moments of levity can become treasured memories and touchstones in a partnership.

Easing Tension: In times of conflict or stress, a shared chuckle can serve as an emotional reset button. It helps to relieve anger and irritation by reminding partners of their affection for one another. Couples can overcome problems more smoothly by finding humor in even the most stressful moments.

Strengthening the Foundation of Friendship

At its root, playfulness strengthens the foundation of friendship in a love relationship.

Enjoying each other's company: Playfulness reminds couples of the simple delight of being together. By participating in enjoyable activities together, partners strengthen the camaraderie that underpins their passionate engagement.

Creating a Strong Partnership: A lighthearted response to life and relationship issues promotes a good partnership. It promotes teamwork, mutual support, and a common sense of purpose. This close bond is necessary for negotiating the complexity of life together.

Chapter 5:Eroticism and the Everyday

Eroticism can be present in everyday life, not just in spectacular gestures or occasional times of passion. In long-term partnerships, the problem is often to maintain desire despite the normal and banal components of daily life. However, when treated with intention and creativity, this routine can be transformed into a canvas for erotic expression. Simple acts such as a lingering touch at breakfast, a meaningful glance across the room, or a shared laugh can inspire a sense of connection and desire. Couples can keep the spark of intimacy alive even on the most mundane of days by finding new methods to inject passion into everyday situations.

The Power of Playfulness.

Playfulness is a potent but frequently ignored aspect of sexuality. In the midst of adulthood, it's easy to forget that humor, teasing, and lightheartedness can be very intimate. Playfulness brings spontaneity and delight into a relationship, establishing an environment in which both partners feel comfortable expressing themselves without fear of being judged. Playfulness, whether via lighthearted banter, exploring with new activities, or simply being funny together, helps to break down barriers and builds a stronger emotional and physical connection. By embracing playfulness, couples can turn daily interactions into opportunities for sensual intimacy.

Cultivating Sensuality in the Ordinary Eroticism does not always require elaborate gestures or special events. Indeed, the simplicity of ordinary existence may provide some of the most profound intimate moments. It's about slowing down and recognizing the small details, such as the touch of your partner's hand as you walk side by side, the way they grin when they see you, or the comfort of being close on a quiet evening. Couples can find passion in their daily lives by paying attention to and thoroughly appreciating these times. It's about being present and making the everyday feel spectacular.

Redefining what intimacy looks like.
Intimacy is more than just physical contact; it also includes emotional connection, shared experiences, and mutual understanding. Everyday activities, such as cooking supper together, conversing over morning coffee, or even doing errands, may become personal experiences if approached with the appropriate perspective. These are moments to connect, exchange thoughts and feelings, and be fully present with one another. When you begin to see intimacy in the smallest details, it becomes easier to sustain that connection, even in the midst of monotony.

Keep Playfulness Alive
Playfulness is an easy method to incorporate sexiness into everyday life. It's about not taking things too seriously and enjoying each other's company. Playfulness, whether in the form of teasing, joking, or doing something stupid together, can help to keep the spark alive. It's a reminder that relationships should be enjoyable, that it's acceptable to let your guard down and simply enjoy being with your spouse. Even the most ordinary situations can be transformed into chances for connection and laughter via play.

Making time for spontaneity.

Routines can get tedious as life gets busier. That is why it is crucial to make time for spontaneity, to surprise each other with small acts of affection, and to occasionally step out of your typical routine. It doesn't have to be anything big—a spontaneous date night, an unexpected praise, or a surprise kiss can work wonders to keep things interesting. Spontaneity keeps the relationship alive and reminds both parties that they're still delighted to be together.

Creating Rituals for Connection

While spontaneity is vital, so are the small rituals that allow you to feel connected. Perhaps it's a morning ritual in which you always share a cup of coffee before beginning your day, or a weekly movie night that you both look forward to. These rituals can serve as touchstones in your relationship, grounding you and reminding you of your link. They do not have to be elaborate—just something consistent that helps you both feel close, regardless of what else is happening on in your lives.

Embracing imperfection

Life is chaotic, and relationships are no exception. Sometimes things don't go as planned, and that's fine. Instead of allowing flaws stand in the way of closeness, embrace them. Laugh at the minor setbacks, be patient with one another, and remember that it is your shortcomings that make your relationship authentic. When you stop striving for perfection, you can make stronger connections and have more honest experiences. True closeness frequently flourishes in these imperfect moments.

**Finding Passion in the Mundane

Find Passion in the Mundane

In long-term partnerships, it's easy to fall into a rut where everything feels overly familiar. The enthusiasm of the early days fades, and what was once fascinating can become ordinary. However, just because life gets more predictable does not mean that passion must disappear. In fact, if we know where to seek, some of the most profound moments of connection can occur every day.

It's about changing your perspective and seeing the beauty in the small things. A shared morning coffee can be more than simply a routine; it can be an opportunity for quiet connection before the day begins. Cooking supper together is more than just putting food on the table; it's an opportunity to collaborate as a group, talk, laugh, and enjoy one other's company. When tackled with the correct perspective, even ordinary jobs such as washing laundry or running errands can become opportunities for connection.

Finding passion in the mundane necessitates being present and intentional. It's about truly seeing your partner, appreciating them, and making time to connect, even in small ways. A simple touch, a kind word, or just spending time together without interruptions can help to maintain that sense of intimacy. These small gestures provide a solid foundation for deeper enthusiasm.

The commonplace does not have to be the adversary of passion; it can be the environment in which passion quietly thrives. When we stop waiting for spectacular gestures and start appreciating the small things in life, we open ourselves up to a long-lasting and genuinely satisfying connection. Passion isn't only about fireworks; it may also mean the continuous, pleasant glow that comes from fully sharing your life with someone.

The Power of Playfulness

Playfulness is one of the most underappreciated but effective instruments for keeping a dynamic relationship. It's easy to get caught up in the seriousness of life—work, bills, responsibilities—but introducing a little humor into your relationship may completely shift the dynamic.

Playfulness encourages laughter, spontaneity, and delight while reminding you not to take things too seriously. Whether it's teasing each other, playing a funny game, or simply messing about, these lighthearted moments allow you to relax and enjoy being together. It's in these moments that you rekindle the carefree spirit that defines the early stages of a relationship.

However, playfulness is more than just having fun; it also strengthens your friendship. When you play with your spouse, you demonstrate that you are at ease, enjoy their company, and respect the connection you have. It's a method to express affection without using words, flirt without being formal, and keep the flame of desire alive.

In a world that might feel oppressive at times, fun can be a welcome relief. It breaks up the routine, relieves tension, and brings you closer together. Making space for play in your relationship builds a foundation of joy and positivity that will help you get through the tough times. So, don't be afraid to be stupid, laugh at yourself, and embrace the fun side of your relationship—it could be the key to keeping your bond intact.

Chapter 6: The Role of Fantasy and Imagination

Fantasy

The human imagination is where the impossible becomes attainable, where our imaginations await their realization, and where our ideas, anxieties, desires, loves, and paranoias exist. It is the world within our world, shaping and being molded by reality. This lesson will discuss the relationship between imagination, fantasy, and reality, as well as the various ways in which fantasy is expressed in the humanities.

Imagination

Imagination permits us to see things that aren't there or haven't been experienced directly. We utilize our imagination to be creative, solve issues, produce ideas, and discover new possibilities. Our imagination enables us to absorb information and organize it in novel and innovative ways. Imagination is an important component of childhood. As children progress from early infancy to primary school, they can utilize their imagination almost like a superpower to investigate ideas and concepts across time and place.

The role of fantasy and imagination in creating reality
'Imagine everyone living in peace.'
Imagination is a uniquely human talent that arises from conscious dreaming to generate new thoughts, images, or concepts that are not visible to awareness or the senses. It involves a set of cognitive processes as a means of producing something from within ourselves, and this enables people to create alternative realities and scenarios that not only include

fantastical creatures and magical worlds, but it also allows people to plan for the future and set goals, engage in hypothetical reasoning, invent and innovate, develop symbols and meanings, design new things, maintain hope, keep faith, and develop the drive to work towards a better world.

Fantasy is derived from the act of visualizing things. It stems from our imagination and the cognitive process of generating unrealistic or implausible mental images or concepts. Fantasy is frequently a response to a psychological need: to develop and invent a solution to a problem, to escape a circumstance, to increase a desire, or to play for relaxation. There are two forms of fantasies: conscious and subconscious, and both articulate with reality.

Importance of Imagination

The power to envision things is inherent in our entire life. It shapes everything we do, think about, and create. It inspires complicated theories, aspirations, and creations in any field, including academia, engineering, and the arts. Finally, imagination permeates all we do, regardless of occupation.

Imagination is essential to invention. So take a time to consider how you may utilize your imagination more efficiently and intentionally.

How to Boost Your Imagination

1. Begin with the aim in mind.

As a leader, you must first understand your goals and have a clear vision of what you want to achieve. As previously said, this is the same path you must take when building a house.

It is critical to have a clear vision of what the ultimate result will look like, unless you are content to simply toss stuff together and see what occurs. It is critical to use creative imagination, as discussed before, particularly the upside-down idea.

While it may seem apparent to start with the end in mind, you'd be shocked how many people don't have a clear picture of what they want to accomplish, let alone how to get there. Instead, they are hindered from achieving their goals by focusing on the roadblocks that stand in their way. You must have a strong, clear vision and, more importantly, understand why that vision is so vital to you.

2. Use both creative and empathic imaginations: This combination is quite effective. When you look back at some of history's great leaders, you'll see that the majority of them had a mission larger than themselves.

Great leaders frequently have a desire for improving the lives of others in addition to their own. Even if they have faced adversity, they can understand what it would be like for those in harsher situations. Consider Mahatma Gandhi, Nelson Mandela, and Mother Teresa; they were all motivated by their empathic imagination.

3. Encourage imagination: It's simpler to discourage than to encourage people's imagination, especially if it's not a part of the workplace culture. It may require considerable guts to challenge a restricted way of thinking. As someone recently told me, "I'd rather have my idea shot down than not say anything and a lesser idea be put forward."
As a team leader, it may be beneficial to read or receive training in the Six Hat Thinking approach. In the corporate world, where reason, truth, facts, and pragmatism reign supreme, I've seen individuals seem concerned and even ashamed when asked to utilize their imagination - as if picturing things is something only children or creative people can do.

The attitude that creativity is somehow inferior to rational thought frequently kills, suppresses, or smothers potential brilliant ideas. Not only does this mindset stifle creative ideas, but it also demonstrates a lack of knowledge of the critical role that imagination plays in human life.

Exploring Desire Safely Establishing Trust and Communication.
A healthy exploration of wants within a relationship is based on trust and open communication:

Building Trust: Trust is the foundation of any healthy relationship and is especially important when exploring desires. Partners must be assured that they can express their dreams without fear of being judged or ridiculed. Establishing a strong sense of trust guarantees that both persons feel comfortable expressing their actual selves.

Open Communication: Transparent and honest communication is essential for safely exploring desires. Couples should talk about their boundaries, comfort levels, and any reservations they might have. Clear discourse helps to avoid misunderstandings and ensures that both partners are on the same page.

Exploring Desires Through Fantasy.

Fantasy can be a safe approach to explore wants without engaging in physical activity.

Fantasy Sharing: Partners can express their fantasies verbally as a means to explore wants without engaging in physical contact. This enables them to assess each other's reactions and comfort levels before determining whether to take any physical action.

Imaginative situations: Engaging in imaginative situations such as storytelling or mental imagery can be a safe approach to explore desires. This strategy allows partners to explore and communicate their desires in a non-threatening setting.

Seeking professional guidance.

Professional advice can offer invaluable assistance and insight: Therapists and counselors: Consulting a therapist or counselor, particularly one who specializes in sexual health and relationships, can help you negotiate complex wants and ensure that both partners feel supported. Professional assistance can offer tools and ideas for safe exploration.

Workshops & Classes: Attending workshops or classes on relationship dynamics and sexual health can provide instruction and a safe environment in which to learn and discuss wants. These venues can offer unique views and practical recommendations on safe exploration.

Celebrating Milestones

Celebrating achievements in exploration can strengthen positive experiences:

Acknowledging Progress Recognizing and praising success, no matter how modest, can perpetuate pleasant feelings and inspire additional investigation. Acknowledging achievements boosts confidence and enjoyment.

Shared rewards: Creating shared prizes for achieving specific goals might make the process more pleasurable. Celebrating together develops a sense of collaboration and achievement.

There are numerous starting locations for your voyage into your own landscapes of desire, and perhaps the exploration will be enjoyable and informative. It may also elicit some uncomfortable feelings or difficulties as you experience and feel the gaps between where you are and where you want to be; you may discover tensions and/or mismatches with a partner or partners; or you may simply come across words, ideas, and thoughts that are new, confusing, exciting, or, perhaps, unsettling.

The trick will be to travel at your own pace. You will need to give these difficulties some space while also giving yourself time to ponder, read, listen, watch, explore, and discuss.

Here are some markers for specific stages of the voyage. It is not an exhaustive list; rather, it serves as a starting point. If you have any more suggestions or questions, please feel free to ask. And, before you begin, please remember that:

***Take things slowly.**
Investigate YOUR wants and desires independently of others. Sharing and discussing with a partner can be enjoyable, but it's important to first consider your own needs and preferences. How difficult is this for you to complete? Be considerate if something is unknown. I still struggle to make time for myself. Writing things down in a notebook, drawing, or simply lying in bed and wondering, watching some videos or looking at images can be a good start.

***Take things slowly.**
Discuss your thoughts with trusted pals. Frame it as a space that you need to share without criticism; if you don't know anyone who can provide this space, look at sites like Pink Therapy.

***Take things slowly.**
Listen to your spouse without judgment, take a break, and remain calm when reflecting on and discussing your own emotions. Really listen to each other and understand that none of you will or should be expected to do anything you are uncomfortable with.
Take breaks as needed, deal with any tough emotions, and get help if necessary.

Questions to Ask Yourself/Things to Consider

1. Exploring Desire

How do you feel about your current levels of desire and sexual activity?

What are your fantasies? Do you have any reoccurring sexual pictures or concepts that you enjoy?

How frequently do you masturbate, and how does it make you feel? Are you reluctant or experimental with yourself? Is it easy for you to set priorities for yourself?

What, if any, pornographic or sexual media do you like seeing, reading, or writing? What are your thoughts on these, and do you feel compelled to share or debate them with others?

What are you most excited about when it comes to sex, desire, and play? How would you convey them to your spouse or partners?

2. Communication, Consent, and Care.

How can you express your feelings regarding sex and desire?

Are you confident in your abilities? If not, how could this be?

How much do you know about?

- Consent - Safe wording

- Boundaries and limitations

- How to speak clearly.

- How to say no, stop something, or cease an interaction. - The importance of aftercare and support. - The relevance of community in the BDSM world.

What kind of help would you like to receive? How able are you to listen reflexively and debate these topics?

How often do you question what you read or watch to ensure that it is appropriate for you and your partner(s)?

3. Meeting people and exploring BDSM.
What do you know about the individual you are considering playing with? The basics you should know are their name, age, sexual health, relationship status, and some backstory.
Do you think they are trustworthy? What is this based on?
Have you met their friends or anyone else who knows them, either inside or outside of the environment in which you met them?
Do you schedule a check-in time for events (for yourself and/or others)? Have you established contingency plans in case you become uncomfortable or want to leave? Have you pondered who to say no to right now?
Are you aware of the end goal of being safe, sane, and consensual?
Do you feel comfortable communicating your discomfort and dealing with a situation that you are unhappy with?
What socials and munches (kink-friendly get-togethers) have you attended? Do you have close, trustworthy friends with whom you can share your hopes, concerns, and fears?

The Benefits of Erotic Creativity
Enhanced Intimacy and Connection
Erotic inventiveness can considerably increase the intimacy and connection between partners:

Emotional Bonding: Creative erotic activities enable partners to share unique and intimate experiences. This shared creation strengthens the emotional link, increasing the sense of closeness and mutual understanding.

Vulnerability: Being erotically creative frequently necessitates a level of vulnerability, which can boost trust. Sharing dreams and desires in a secure atmosphere allows couples to expose aspects of themselves that they might otherwise hide, resulting in a closer relationship.

Revitalizing Passion

Bringing creativity into the sensual world can rekindle desire and excitement:

Breaking typical: Erotic inventiveness helps to break the monotony of typical sexual acts, adding freshness and excitement to the relationship. New experiences can reignite the spark and keep the expectation and desire alive.

Exploring New avenues: Creative erotic activities provide new opportunities for sexual discovery. Partners can uncover new sources of pleasure and excitement by role-playing, trying out new props, or experimenting with other surroundings.

Personal Development and Self-Discovery

Erotic creativity can promote personal development and self-discovery:

Understanding Desires: Experimenting with erotic creativity can help people and couples better understand their own desires and preferences. This self-awareness can result in more gratifying and fulfilling sexual encounters.

Confidence Boosting: Successfully discovering and expressing erotic creativity can increase self-esteem and confidence. Feeling at ease and accepted in one's sexual expression promotes high self-esteem and a more confident attitude to intimacy.

Encourage Playfulness and Fun.
Erotic creativity promotes a sense of playfulness and enjoyment in the relationship.
Light-Hearted Exploration: Approaching sensual creation with a fun attitude helps relieve stress and anxiety. This lighthearted exploration makes sexual acts more engaging and less daunting, resulting in a good and fun environment.
Joy and Laughter: Incorporating humor and playfulness into sensual activities can result in delight and laughter, increasing the whole experience. This shared excitement increases the emotional tie, leading to a happier and more meaningful relationship.

Let's Talk About Sex and Creativity.
Sex is creative.
Sex, whether with someone you like or alone, necessitates both setting limits and letting go of control, something poets and mystics have waxed lyrical about for decades (but said much better).

Sexual energy may fuel inspiration and enthusiasm, and when harnessed and correctly channeled, "is a pleasurable and powerful means to motivate us creatively,"

Sex is also the ultimate source of life. It is the catalyst for procreation. "But even if you choose not to procreate or if you engage in sex that would never lead to conception, you are co-creating an experience with another human being."

Sex is typically shrouded in shame. Or we discuss it from a performance perspective. There are numbers, roles, and goals to accomplish. We don't talk about the benefits of sex connection: how intimacy creates a moment together, how wonderful sex helps you communicate what you want and don't want.
We never learn that it may be a channel for creativity.

***Tap into the erotic**.
"The erotic is a measure between the beginnings of our sense of self and the chaos of our most intense emotions. It is an inward sense of satisfaction that, once experienced, we know we can strive for. We can expect nothing less of ourselves after experiencing the depths of this depth of feeling and realizing its strength, in honor and self-respect."

Tapping into this deep well of desire, letting go of control and staying focused while also relaxing into sensations of boundless riches and power, is not only a lovely feeling—one that every person should be able to have—but also freeing. We let go of our concerns, comparisons, and uncertainties, which is an excellent beginning place for diving into creation.

Whatever you do, don't include sex in your work.
No matter how much sexual energy you utilize to harness creative strength, filthy sex is not acceptable in your creative endeavors. Exploring sexual topics too clearly is the quickest

way to lose representation, the green light (definitely not the red light), and money.

But tap into your inner Eros, the universal sense of great desire, and say yes to whatever you want, even if only for ten minutes. And see where the creative spirit leads you.

Chapter 7: Communicating in the Language of Eroticism

Two languages of closeness
Modern partnerships require self-disclosure, emotional sharing, and active listening (nonjudgmental, validating, etc.). We want to feel understood, and we expect our partners to share just as much as we do. However, conversing is not the only (or even the best) way to cultivate intimacy. There are two methods for communicating intimacy: vocally and physically.

*Verbal Communication: Women's Arena
Women's personal language is mostly verbal, as women have historically lacked access to authority. Instead, they improved their relationship-building skills. Even today, girls are taught how to develop relationship skills.

The emphasis on talking as the primary technique of establishing intimacy emerged at the same time that women gained economic independence. As women became less financially dependent on their husbands, they had higher expectations of marriage. Women sought emotional connection in their relationships, and because they were so at ease with verbal communication, they used it to promote intimacy.

*Physical Communication: Men's Arena.
However, men have not been socialized in the same way as women. Men are taught to compete and perform with confidence, fearlessness, and invulnerability. For men, expressing feelings is frequently not just not part of the

curriculum, but actively discouraged. Attempting to create closeness just through speech can result in guys trying to cram a language they do not speak.

Some of the limitations on men's socialization have led them to express themselves and communicate through their bodies. Most people are aware of the classic violent male sexuality, but few understand that sexuality can also elicit tenderness. Sex is a nonverbal mode of communication.

Conflict between communication approaches.
People who value verbal communication find it difficult to realize that there are other ways to express intimacy. This results in the talker striving to persuade the non-talker to switch languages. However, nonverbal communication can be just as important as verbal communication, especially when the speaker is learning a second language.

Eddie, for example, was dumped by a number of women because he failed to communicate. They assumed he was fearful of committing and unable to be open about himself. He married a Japanese woman who spoke little English (he did not know Japanese). They couldn't communicate, so they conveyed their love in other ways, such as by showing each other art, cleaning each other, and cooking for each other. They communicated, but not via talking.

Utilizing Verbal and Nonverbal Communication.

Erotic impulses are expressed through both verbal and nonverbal communication.

*Verbal Communication: Using words to express wishes, fantasies, and boundaries is both direct and powerful. Discussing these subjects openly allows partners to handle their sexual relationship with clarity and confidence.

*Nonverbal Cues: Body language, touch, and eye contact are excellent nonverbal clues for communicating erotic desires and boundaries. Being sensitive to these cues allows partners to respond appropriately and improves the overall sensual experience.

Overcoming Barriers to Erotic Communication

Addressing and overcoming barriers to erotic communication is crucial for a healthy partnership.

*Addressing Shame and Guilt: Feelings of shame or guilt surrounding sexual impulses might inhibit frank discourse. Partners should work together to create a supportive environment where these feelings can be discussed and resolved.

Cultural and social norms can influence how people discuss sex. Understanding these pressures and working to overcome them may lead to more open and honest erotic conversations.

The Importance of Honest Conversations

Developing trust and closeness.

Honest conversations are vital for building trust and intimacy in a relationship.

*Creating a safe space: When partners communicate openly, they create a safe environment in which both parties feel comfortable expressing their true personalities. This safety fosters a deeper emotional connection and greater attachment.

*Fostering Vulnerability: Honest interactions encourage vulnerability by allowing partners to disclose their most intimate thoughts, concerns, and desires. This openness develops closeness and allows partners to understand each other on a deeper level.

Enhancing Relationship Satisfaction.

Honest communication leads directly to relationship fulfillment.

*Alignment of expectations: Clear and honest communication ensures that both partners understand their needs, expectations, and boundaries. This alignment helps to prevent misunderstandings and confrontations.

*Addressing Issues Promptly: When partners are honest, they may address difficulties and concerns before they become more serious. This proactive approach encourages a harmonious and rewarding connection.

Promoting Personal Growth

Honest interactions can promote personal development and self-awareness.

*Self-Reflection: Engaging in honest conversations encourages self-reflection. Partners who communicate openly are more likely to reflect on their own behaviors, motivations, and desires, leading to personal growth.

*Learning and Adapting: Your partner's honest feedback can help you identify areas for improvement. Positive feedback helps people grow, adapt, and become better partners.

Facilitating Mutual Understanding.

Honest conversations improve mutual understanding significantly.

Honest communication can help to clear up misunderstandings. Partners who communicate openly can discuss and resolve any misunderstandings, resulting in a clear and accurate comprehension.

Honest relationships foster understanding and compassion. When couples communicate openly about their experiences and emotions, they develop a stronger understanding and compassion for one another's points of view.

Enhancing Sexual Satisfaction

Honest conversations about sex can significantly increase sexual satisfaction:

*Expressing desires: The honest presentation of sexual desires and preferences guarantees that both partners' needs are addressed. Honest discussions about what each partner appreciates result in more meaningful and gratifying experiences.

*Discussing Boundaries: Honest conversations discussing limitations are vital for sustaining comfort and consent during sexual engagement. This dialog makes partners feel at ease and respected, which boosts overall sexual pleasure.

Finally, open and honest communication is vital for team development. They promote trust, foster an open culture, resolve conflicts, contribute to individual and team development, and improve communication skills. Teams that encourage honest interactions create an environment in which members feel heard, respected, and valued. The only way ahead is for everyone to contribute honestly, regardless of rank or status. All you have to do is make the conscious decision to act with integrity and put your best foot forward every day, in every situation. Being able to attain your best is highly motivating for all discussion partners. With more transparency and integrity, honest conversations start having ripple effects on the culture.

Overcome Shame and Guilt
Understanding the Roots of Shame and Guilt.
Identifying the sources of shame and guilt is the first step toward overcoming them.

Cultural and societal standards regarding sexuality and relationships have a significant impact on many feelings of shame and guilt. Understanding these consequences enables individuals to define their emotions and begin to challenge them.

Personal Experience: Feelings of shame and guilt can be influenced by past experiences such as trauma, upbringing, and relationships. Reflecting on these events assists people to recognize and address the roots of their emotions.

What are guilt and shame?
Guilt and shame are sometimes portrayed as the same emotions, but there are some crucial distinctions.

Guilt is the admittance that we have done something wrong, but it does not define who we are as individuals. Someone who is suffering guilt can acknowledge their wonderful traits while still viewing themselves positively.

Shame is the belief that we have done something wrong, which makes us horrible people. Someone who feels ashamed may be unable to recognize their positive qualities or see themselves in a good light.

Recognizing shame
We can experience and recognize shame in a variety of ways, including physical, emotional, and behavioral cues. Recognizing when you feel ashamed is the first step toward managing that feeling so that it does not become harmful.

Acknowledging and Accepting Feelings
Acknowledging and accepting feelings of shame and guilt is essential for overcoming them:
- Self-Awareness: Developing self-awareness involves recognizing and acknowledging feelings of shame and guilt when they arise. This awareness is the first step towards addressing and managing these emotions.

- Acceptance Without Judgment: Accepting these feelings without self-judgment is crucial. Understanding that these emotions are natural and common helps reduce their power and allows for a more compassionate self-view.

Practicing Self-Compassion

Self-compassion is a powerful tool for overcoming shame and guilt:

- Kindness to Oneself: Treating oneself with kindness and understanding, as one would a friend, helps mitigate the harshness of shame and guilt. Self-compassion involves recognizing one's humanity and accepting imperfections.
- Reframing Negative Self-Talk: Reframing negative self-talk into positive or neutral statements can significantly reduce feelings of shame and guilt. This practice involves challenging and changing the internal narrative to be more supportive and forgiving.

Seeking Support

Seeking support from others can provide valuable perspectives and encouragement:

- Talking to a Trusted Friend or Partner: Sharing feelings of shame and guilt with a trusted friend or partner can provide relief and support. Loved ones can offer empathy, understanding, and reassurance.
- Professional Help: Therapy or counseling can be highly effective in addressing deep-seated shame and guilt. A professional can help individuals explore the roots of

these emotions and develop strategies for overcoming them.

Chapter 8: When Love Meets Desire

The Interplay Between Love and Desire

Understanding the dynamic interaction between love and desire is vital for a satisfying relationship.

- Emotional Connection: Deep compassion, care, and mutual respect are common characteristics of love. In contrast, desire is fueled by physical attraction and sexual need. Balancing these two characteristics can result in a truly fulfilling relationship.
- Balancing Acts: Love and desire can sometimes seem at conflict with one another. Love craves consistency and comfort, whereas desire lives on novelty and excitement. Successful partnerships find a way to balance these competing impulses, allowing love and desire to exist in harmony.

Managing Conflicts of Love and Desire

Conflicts between love and desire can occur, but they can be skillfully managed.

- Acknowledging Differences: Recognizing that variances in sexual desire and emotional needs are normal might help avert conflict. Understanding that each partner's level of desire varies at different times promotes empathy and patience.
- Finding compromises: Finding compromises that meet both emotional and physical needs is critical. This may entail negotiating the number, timing, and sorts of intimate actions to ensure that both partners are satisfied.

The Role of Individual Growth

Individual growth and self-awareness help to maintain a healthy balance of love and desire.

- Personal Development: Supporting one another's personal development and growth develops a sense of individuality and self-confidence. This personal fulfillment might increase overall desire and attraction.
- Mutual Respect: Respecting each other's autonomy and individuality within the partnership fosters both love and desire. Mutual respect promotes a positive dynamic in which both partners feel valued and respected.

Cultivating emotional and physical intimacy

Integrating love and desire requires cultivating both emotional and physical connection.

- Emotional Intimacy: Strengthening the tie of love by engaging in meaningful conversations, sharing values, and providing mutual support. Emotional connection increases total relationship satisfaction.
- Physical closeness: Regular physical closeness, including sexual activity, strengthens the bond and fuels desire. Exploring one other's bodies and sharing intimate moments strengthens the physical bond in the partnership.

Overcoming Challenges Together

Facing obstacles together increases the bond between love and desire.

- Supportive Partnership: Showing support and empathy during difficult times strengthens the emotional tie. This connection promotes resilience and assures that love and desire can withstand any storm.
- Problem-Solving: Approaching difficulties as a group and devising solutions jointly enhances the bond. Collaborative problem-solving builds trust and strengthens the emotional connection, which increases desire.

Maintaining sexual chemistry over time and prioritizing intimacy.

To maintain sexual chemistry, you must prioritize connection in your relationship.

- Scheduled intimacy: While spontaneity is vital, arranging frequent intimate moments ensures that both spouses make time to connect. This does not dampen the enthusiasm, but rather ensures that closeness is always prioritized.
- Quality Over Quantity: Concentrate on the quality of personal meetings rather than their frequency. Meaningful, engaged encounters can be more rewarding than a larger number of disconnected experiences.

Keep the spark alive.

Keeping the initial excitement alive requires consistent effort and creativity.

- Exploring Fantasies: Sharing and exploring each other's fantasies can offer additional depth to your sexual relationship. This openness has the potential to revive enthusiasm and curiosity.

- Trying new things: Introducing new activities, positions, or settings can help keep things interesting. Trying new activities together fosters a sense of adventure and freshness.

Open Communication

Open conversation about sexual desires and demands is critical.

- Expressing Needs: Partners should feel free to share their sexual needs and aspirations without fear of criticism. Honest interactions guarantee that both partners' needs are acknowledged and met.
- Active Listening: Paying attention to your partner's desires and concerns promotes a stronger connection and understanding. This mutual respect promotes intimacy and chemistry.

Physical Affection

Regular physical affection outside of sexual activity promotes connection.

- Touch & Cuddling: Simple acts of touch, like holding hands, embracing, and cuddling, help to strengthen physical connection and closeness. These gestures keep the spark alive.
- Nonsexual Intimacy: Non-sexual physical contact, such as massages or stroking, preserves a physical connection and can frequently lead to increased sexual chemistry.

Playfulness and Humor

Incorporating playfulness and comedy into your relationship might improve sexual chemistry.

Flirting, teasing, and playful exchanges can help keep the relationship alive and exciting. This playfulness promotes a lighthearted connection, which improves sexual chemistry.

- Laughter: Sharing laughter and humor helps to decrease stress and enhances relationships. A partnership that combines joy and humor is more likely to retain sexual chemistry over time.

-

Seeking Professional Help.

When necessary, obtaining expert assistance can resolve sexual chemistry issues:

Couples therapy, sometimes known as sex therapy, can assist partners in overcoming obstacles and improving their sexual relationship. A therapist can provide tools and ways to improve intimacy.

- Medicinal Advice: Consultation with a medical practitioner about sexual health issues can help address physical limitations to maintaining sexual chemistry. This can involve hormonal shifts, sexual dysfunction, and other health issues.

Strategies for Rekindling Passion

Open Communication

Rekindling passion requires effective communication.

Expressing Desires: Partners should talk honestly about their sexual aspirations. This candor promotes intimacy and has the potential to reignite the spark.

Active Listening: Actively listening to each other's wants and concerns aids in identifying and addressing any underlying issues that may be dampening passion.

Physical intimacy and touch

Physical touch and compassion are essential for sustaining and rekindling romance.

Non-Sexual Touch: Holding hands, embracing, or snuggling can all help to increase physical affection. These actions can foster a stronger emotional and physical closeness.

Massage and Sensual Activities: Massages and other forms of sensuous touch between partners can increase intimacy and desire.

Prioritizing our time together

Spending quality time together fosters connection and passion.

Scheduled Date Nights: Regular date nights guarantee that you focus your relationship despite your hectic schedule. These designated times for connecting might renew the spark.

Technology-Free Time: Spend time together away from technology. This undivided focus promotes deeper connections and intimacy.

Enhancing Emotional Intimacy

Building emotional intimacy improves the total connection, making it easier to rekindle passion.

Meaningful Conversation: Have deep, meaningful conversations about your dreams, anxieties, and goals. Sharing at this level strengthens emotional ties.

Shared Experiences: Take part in activities that foster shared experiences and memories, such as attending a class together or collaborating on a project. This shared time and effort can lead to greater emotional connection.

Romantic gestures.

Small romantic gestures can have a significant impact on reigniting passion:

Surprise and spontaneity: Surprise your sweetheart with thoughtful gestures such as a handwritten note, an unexpected date, or a small gift. These expressions of love demonstrate appreciation and might rekindle the spark.

Affirmations and compliments: Express your affection and admiration on a regular basis using affirmations and compliments. These positive reinforcements help your spouse feel cherished and desired.

Chapter 9: Cultural Influences on Sexuality

Impact of Cultural Norms

Cultural norms influence our attitudes and behaviors regarding sexuality in major ways. Social norms frequently affect what constitutes suitable or inappropriate sexual activity. For example, in certain cultures, publicly discussing sex is taboo, yet in others, it is a common topic of conversation. Traditional gender norms can also play a role, with differing expectations placed on men and women in terms of sexual conduct and wants. These cultural conventions shape how we see ourselves and our partners sexually.

The Function of Religion and Morality

Religious and moral beliefs frequently influence sexual attitudes. Many religions have unique teachings on sexuality that encourage some acts while condemning others. These teachings can have a significant impact on our sexual beliefs and conduct, sometimes leading to feelings of guilt or shame when our impulses collide with these moral guidelines. For example, some religious systems may call for abstinence before marriage, which might influence how people approach their sexual interactions.

Media and Sexuality

The media has a strong influence on our sexual conventions and habits. How sex and sexuality are represented in films, television shows, and commercials can influence cultural attitudes and individual perceptions. Positive depictions can encourage healthy views regarding sex, whereas bad or unrealistic portrayals might lead to distorted expectations.

Pornography, in particular, can have a substantial impact by shaping attitudes toward body image, sexual practices, and relationship dynamics.

Historical Perspectives.

Historical factors also influence our attitudes toward sexuality. Cultural upheavals, such as the sexual revolution of the 1960s, have gradually changed sexual standards and behaviors. Understanding these transitions helps us better understand modern attitudes regarding sexuality. Recognizing the historical oppression of specific groups, such as women and LGBTQ+ people, is also critical for understanding current sexual norms and battles.

Education & Sexuality

Sex education varies substantially across cultures and has a considerable impact on sexual behavior and attitudes. In some cultures, thorough sex education is provided, which encourages healthy sexual attitudes and helps to minimize teenage pregnancy and STI rates. Individuals in cultures where abstinence-only instruction is common may be less equipped to make educated decisions about their sexual health, increasing the chance of poor outcomes.

The Influence of Technology

Technology has significantly altered sexual conventions and practices. The proliferation of online dating sites has altered how people meet and build relationships, frequently altering sexual practices and expectations. Additionally, digital communication forms such as sexting and cybersex have grown in popularity, providing new methods for people to express their sexuality and sustain intimacy even from a distance.

Legal and Political Context

The legal and political environments can influence sexual norms and rights. Laws governing sexual activity, such as the legality of same-sex relationships or access to contraception and abortion, reflect and shape cultural attitudes toward sexuality. Political action can drive change in these areas, with movements pushing for LGBTQ+ rights, gender equality, and sexual health having a significant impact on cultural beliefs and legal norms.

Intersection of Sexuality and Identity

Sexuality is intimately linked to our personal and societal identities. Cultural attitudes about various sexual orientations and gender identities fluctuate significantly, influencing how people express themselves and their mental health. Intersectionality, or the idea that multiple dimensions of identification, such as race, ethnicity, and socioeconomic class, intersect and influence sexuality experiences, is critical for understanding the wide range of issues people confront.

Overcoming Cultural Barriers

Identifying and overcoming cultural barriers to healthy sexuality is critical. Being culturally sensitive and respectful of other customs and values promotes understanding while reducing conflict. Promoting sexual education and campaigning for sexual rights can help break down these barriers, empowering people to make informed decisions and creating a more inclusive society.

Embracing Culture Change

Cultural ideas toward sexuality are always changing. Accepting these changes is part of cultural progress. As individuals and cultures, responding to these changes encourages healthy and inclusive attitudes toward sexuality. Actively encouraging good change, questioning harmful conventions, pushing for rights, and teaching future generations are all methods to create a healthier, more welcoming environment for everybody.

How Society Shapes Our Desires

Cultural norms and expectations.

Society has a strong influence on our desires, frequently through cultural norms and expectations that we experience at a young age. These standards define what is acceptable or taboo in our sexual and romantic life. For example, many cultures place a high value on marriage and having children, which influences how people perceive relationships and sexual activity. These cultural norms can influence anything from who we consider attractive to how we express our sexuality.

Media & Popular Culture

The media we consume has a strong influence on our wants. Movies, television shows, ads, and social media frequently present romanticized depictions of love, sex, and relationships. These depictions might develop false expectations and desires based on fantasy rather than reality. For example, the presence of ideal bodies and romantic fairy tales can lead to individuals desiring similar experiences, often leaving them disappointed with their own lives when they don't meet expectations.

Gender Roles and Stereotypes

Desires are heavily influenced by traditional gender norms and prejudices. Men and women are frequently socialized differently, with differing expectations for their sexual behavior and wants. Men may be pushed to be forceful and pursue several sexual partners, whilst women may be trained to value emotional connection and modesty. These prejudices can limit people's comprehension of their own aspirations, resulting in internal conflicts.

Peer Influence

Our peers might have a tremendous impact on our desires. People may conform to their social groups' sexual standards and practices out of a desire to fit in and be liked. Adolescents and young adults, in particular, may feel pressured to engage in certain sexual activities or adopt specific attitudes regarding sex in order to receive approval from their peers. Peer pressure can shape desires that are more aligned with group norms than with individual preferences.

Family and Upbringing

Our family environment and upbringing shape how we perceive and experience desire. Parents and caregivers' views and attitudes on sex, relationships, and love can have a significant impact on our wants. Families that freely discuss these issues can promote a healthy perspective of sexuality, whereas those that avoid or stigmatize them can lead to uncertainty and shame about natural impulses.

Religious and Moral Values

Religion and moral ideals frequently give a framework for comprehending and managing impulses. Many religions have specific norms for sexual behavior, which might impact what people believe is appropriate and immoral to desire. These moral ideals can either match with human wants, offering a sense of clarity, or contradict them, resulting in emotions of guilt and shame.

Economic and Social Status

Our economic and social status can influence our preferences. Access to resources, education, and social chances can all have an impact on the types of relationships and goals we pursue. For example, people from wealthier origins may have different expectations and ambitions than those from less privileged backgrounds. Social position can also influence how free one feels in expressing their wishes.

Intersectionality

Our wants are also shaped by the junction of many facets of our identity, such as race, ethnicity, sexual orientation, and gender identity. Each of these dimensions has the potential to influence our experiences and wants in unique ways. For example, a gay person of color's experiences may differ significantly from those of a heterosexual, white person, resulting in various understandings and displays of desire.

Personal Experience and Trauma

Finally, personal events and trauma have a significant impact on our desires. Positive experiences can strengthen healthy desires, but unpleasant experiences like abuse or rejection can distort or repress them. Understanding and treating these experiences is critical for having a positive connection with one's desires.

Embracing authentic desires

Navigating the various ways in which culture shapes our aspirations can be tough. It takes self-reflection and, in some cases, boldness to question conventional standards. Embracing true desires is discovering and accepting what actually makes you happy, outside of society expectations and pressures. It entails identifying and understanding your own needs and desires, as well as striking a balance between society pressures and personal authenticity.

Breaking Free from Normative Expectations

- Understanding Normative Expectations

Normative expectations are the unwritten rules society imposes on us about how we should behave, think, and feel. They cover everything from career choices to relationships, and they often shape our lives in profound ways without us even realizing it. Breaking free from these expectations can be challenging but incredibly liberating.

- Challenging Gender Roles

Traditional gender roles are some of the most pervasive normative expectations. They dictate how men and women should behave, often limiting opportunities and self-expression. Challenging these roles means rejecting stereotypes and embracing a more fluid understanding of gender. This might involve pursuing careers or hobbies traditionally associated with the opposite gender, or expressing yourself in ways that feel true to you, regardless of societal expectations.

- Pursuing Authentic Relationships

Normative expectations also shape our relationships, from whom we date to how we interact with our partners. Breaking free involves pursuing relationships that align with your values and desires, rather than those society deems appropriate. This might mean embracing non-traditional relationship structures, such as polyamory or choosing not to marry or have children. Authentic relationships are built on mutual respect, understanding, and a shared commitment to each other's well-being.

- Overcoming Fear of Judgment

Fear of judgment is a significant barrier to breaking free from normative expectations. Worrying about what others will think can keep us trapped in lives that don't truly satisfy us. Overcoming this fear involves building self-confidence and finding a supportive community. Surround yourself with people who respect and encourage your individuality, and practice self-compassion to combat negative self-talk.

- Redefining Success

Society often has a narrow definition of success, typically centered around wealth, status, and conventional achievements. Redefining success on your own terms means identifying what truly matters to you. This could be happiness, fulfillment, meaningful relationships, or personal growth. By setting your own standards for success, you can pursue a life that feels rich and rewarding, regardless of societal pressures.

- Taking Small Steps

Breaking free from normative expectations doesn't happen overnight. It involves taking small, deliberate steps toward living more authentically. Start by making minor changes in your daily life that align more closely with your true self. Gradually, these small actions will build momentum, leading to more significant changes and a greater sense of freedom.

- Seeking Professional Support

Sometimes, the pressure to conform can be overwhelming, and professional support can be invaluable. Therapists, coaches, and mentors can provide guidance and encouragement as you navigate the process of breaking free. They can help you explore your identity, set realistic goals, and develop strategies to overcome obstacles.

- Celebrating Your Journey

Breaking free from normative expectations is a journey worth celebrating. Each step you take toward living authentically is an achievement. Acknowledge and celebrate these milestones, no matter how small they may seem. Celebrating your progress reinforces your commitment to your true self and encourages you to continue on this liberating path.

- Inspiring Others

As you break free and embrace your individuality, you may find that you inspire others to do the same. Your courage and authenticity can encourage those around you to question societal norms and pursue their true desires. By living authentically, you contribute to a more inclusive and accepting society where everyone feels free to be themselves.

- Continuing the Journey

Breaking free from normative expectations is an ongoing process. As society evolves, new norms and expectations will emerge. Continuously reassessing and realigning your life with your true self is essential. Stay curious, open-minded, and committed to personal growth, and you will continue to thrive outside the confines of societal expectations.

Chapter 10: Conclusion: The Art of Keeping Desire Alive

Understanding the Challenge

Keeping desire alive in long-term relationships is one of the greatest challenges couples face. The initial spark of attraction and passion often fades as familiarity and routine set in. However, maintaining desire is essential for a fulfilling and dynamic relationship. It's not just about sexual attraction but also about sustaining emotional and intellectual connection.

☐ Embracing Change

One of the keys to keeping desire alive is embracing change. People grow and evolve over time, and so do their needs and desires. Rather than fearing these changes, couples should see them as opportunities to rediscover each other. Regularly exploring new activities, hobbies, and interests together can help keep the relationship fresh and exciting.

☐ Prioritizing Intimacy

Intimacy goes beyond physical closeness; it includes emotional and psychological connection. Prioritizing intimacy means making time for each other despite busy schedules. This could be through regular date nights, meaningful conversations, or simply spending quality time together without distractions. It's about being present and attentive to each other's needs and feelings.

☐ Communicating openly

Open and honest communication is crucial for maintaining desire. Couples should feel comfortable discussing their desires, fantasies, and boundaries. This openness fosters a deeper understanding and trust, allowing both partners to feel safe and valued. Addressing issues and conflicts as they arise, rather than letting them fester, helps prevent resentment and keeps the relationship healthy.

☐ Cultivating Playfulness

Playfulness is often overlooked in adult relationships, yet it's a powerful tool for maintaining desire. Bringing a sense of fun and spontaneity into the relationship can reignite the spark. This could be through playful teasing, surprising each other with small gestures, or experimenting with new things in the bedroom. Playfulness keeps the relationship light-hearted and enjoyable.

☐ Balancing Independence and Togetherness

Maintaining desire requires a balance between independence and togetherness. While spending quality time together is important, it's equally vital for each partner to have their own space and interests. Encouraging each other's personal growth and respecting individual autonomy can prevent feelings of suffocation and boredom. A healthy balance allows both partners to bring new experiences and energy into the relationship.

☐ Keeping the Mystery Alive

Desire thrives on a sense of mystery and novelty. Even in long-term relationships, maintaining an element of mystery can keep the excitement alive. This doesn't mean hiding things from each other, but rather, continuously finding ways to surprise and intrigue your partner. It could be through unexpected acts of kindness, learning new skills, or sharing hidden talents.

☐ Nurturing Emotional Connection

Emotional connection is the foundation of lasting desire. Couples should nurture this connection by being emotionally available and supportive. Sharing dreams, fears, and vulnerabilities can deepen the bond and enhance intimacy. Acts of empathy, understanding, and appreciation go a long way in maintaining a strong emotional connection.

☐ Investing in Personal Well-being

Personal well-being directly impacts the quality of the relationship. Taking care of oneself physically, mentally, and emotionally ensures that you can bring your best self into the relationship. Regular exercise, healthy eating, mindfulness practices, and pursuing personal passions contribute to overall happiness and vitality, which in turn, keeps the relationship vibrant.

☐ Seeking Professional Help When Needed

There is no shame in seeking professional help to maintain desire in a relationship. Therapists and counselors can provide valuable insights and strategies to navigate challenges. Whether it's dealing with intimacy issues, communication problems, or past traumas, professional guidance can help couples strengthen their bond and rekindle desire.

☐ Celebrating Milestones

Celebrating milestones, both big and small, is essential for keeping desire alive. Acknowledging anniversaries, achievements, and shared memories reinforces the bond and reminds couples of their journey together. These celebrations don't have to be extravagant; it's the act of recognition and appreciation that matters most.

☐ Commitment to Growth

Finally, keeping desire alive requires a commitment to growth. Relationships are dynamic, and maintaining desire is an ongoing process. Couples should continually strive to learn more about each other, adapt to changes, and work towards mutual goals. This commitment to growth fosters a resilient and enduring desire that can withstand the test of time.

☐

Conclusion

The art of keeping desire alive is a multifaceted endeavor that involves embracing change, prioritizing intimacy, communicating openly, and maintaining a balance between independence and togetherness. By nurturing emotional connection, investing in personal well-being, seeking professional help when needed, celebrating milestones, and committing to continuous growth, couples can sustain a vibrant and passionate relationship. It's about creating a dynamic partnership where both individuals feel valued, understood, and deeply connected, ensuring that desire remains a vital and enduring part of their shared journey.

Embracing the Ongoing Journey

☐ The Ever-Evolving Relationship

Relationships are not static; they are dynamic and constantly evolving. As individuals, we grow and change over time, and so do our relationships. Embracing this ongoing journey means recognizing that change is natural and necessary for a healthy partnership. It's about understanding that the relationship you started with will inevitably transform, and that's a positive thing.

☐ Accepting Growth and Change

One of the first steps in embracing the journey is accepting that growth and change are part of life. Personal growth can be exciting and sometimes daunting, but it enriches our lives and relationships. As partners grow individually, they bring new experiences, perspectives, and strengths into the relationship. Embracing this growth rather than resisting it can lead to a more fulfilling and dynamic partnership.

☐ Continuous Learning and Discovery

In long-term relationships, there is always something new to learn about your partner. People are complex and multifaceted, and even after years together, there are aspects of each other that remain undiscovered. Maintaining curiosity about your partner and being open to learning new things about them keeps the relationship fresh and engaging. This continuous discovery fosters deeper understanding and connection.

☐ Setting and Revisiting Goals

Setting goals together is an important part of the ongoing journey. Whether they are personal goals, career ambitions, or dreams for the future, having shared goals can unite partners and provide a sense of purpose. It's also crucial to revisit and adjust these goals as life progresses. Regularly checking in on each other's aspirations and aligning them with the relationship's direction helps ensure that both partners feel supported and valued.

☐ Celebrating Milestones

Celebrating milestones is a way to honor the journey you've shared. These milestones can be anniversaries, personal achievements, or overcoming challenges together. Taking time to celebrate reinforces the bond and reminds couples of their shared history and accomplishments. These moments of recognition and joy contribute to a positive and enduring relationship.

☐ Practicing Patience and Compassion

Patience and compassion are essential qualities in a long-term relationship. Understanding that both partners will make mistakes and face difficulties allows for a more forgiving and supportive environment. Practicing compassion means empathizing with each other's struggles and being patient as you both grow and learn. This creates a safe space for vulnerability and honesty.

☐ Committing to the Journey

Embracing the journey requires a commitment to the relationship and to each other. It's about being willing to put in the effort to maintain and nurture the relationship, even when faced with challenges. This commitment involves a shared vision for the future and a dedication to working through difficulties together. It's about seeing the relationship as a lifelong journey that evolves and grows over time.

☐ Finding Joy in the Everyday

Finally, embracing the journey means finding joy in the everyday moments. It's about appreciating the small, mundane aspects of life that you share with your partner. These moments of connection, laughter, and companionship are what make the journey meaningful. By finding joy in the ordinary, couples can build a strong foundation of happiness and contentment.

In conclusion, embracing the ongoing journey in a relationship involves accepting growth and change, continuously learning about each other, adapting to life's changes, and nurturing emotional intimacy. It requires patience, compassion, and a commitment to maintaining the spark and mutual respect. By celebrating milestones and finding joy in everyday moments, couples can create a fulfilling and enduring partnership that thrives through all phases of life.

The Future of Intimacy and Eroticism

☐ Technological Advancements and Their Impact

As technology continues to advance, its impact on intimacy and eroticism is becoming increasingly profound. Virtual reality (VR), augmented reality (AR), and artificial intelligence (AI) are beginning to transform how people experience and explore their desires. VR and AR can create immersive experiences that allow couples to connect in new ways, even when physically apart. AI-driven sex robots and virtual partners are pushing the boundaries of what constitutes a relationship, providing companionship and sexual gratification in ways that were once purely science fiction.

☐ Redefining Relationships

The definition of relationships is evolving. The traditional monogamous relationship is no longer the only model people aspire to. Polyamory, open relationships, and other non-traditional structures are becoming more accepted and explored. This shift allows individuals to tailor their relationships to better fit their needs and desires, leading to more honest and fulfilling connections. The future of intimacy will likely see a continued diversification of relationship models, as people seek to find what works best for them without the constraints of societal norms.

☐ The Role of Social Media

Social media plays a significant role in shaping perceptions of intimacy and eroticism. Platforms like Instagram, TikTok, and OnlyFans allow individuals to express their sexuality more openly and connect with others who share similar interests. While this can promote a more inclusive and accepting environment, it also raises questions about privacy and the commodification of intimacy. Navigating these platforms responsibly will be crucial as they continue to influence how people experience and perceive eroticism.

☐ Shifting Gender Norms and Sexuality

Gender norms and perceptions of sexuality are shifting, leading to a more fluid understanding of both. The binary view of gender is being challenged, with more people identifying as non-binary, genderqueer, or fluid. This shift is also affecting how people experience intimacy and eroticism. As society becomes more accepting of diverse gender identities and sexual orientations, individuals feel freer to explore their desires without fear of judgment. The future promises a broader acceptance of various forms of intimacy and a celebration of individuality in eroticism.

☐ Mental Health and Intimacy

The connection between mental health and intimacy is gaining more recognition. Understanding that mental well-being significantly impacts one's ability to experience and enjoy intimate relationships is crucial. Future approaches to intimacy will likely place greater emphasis on mental health, encouraging individuals to seek therapy or counseling to address issues that may hinder their ability to connect with others. This holistic approach can lead to healthier, more fulfilling relationships.

☐ The Intersection of Health and Technology

Advancements in health and technology are intersecting in ways that enhance intimacy and sexual health. Innovations in sexual health products, such as wearable tech that monitors physiological responses, can provide insights into sexual well-being and help improve experiences. Additionally, telehealth services are making it easier for individuals to access sexual health resources and support, ensuring that people can take proactive steps in maintaining their sexual health.

☐ The Importance of Education

Comprehensive sex education is critical for the future of intimacy and eroticism. Providing accurate, inclusive, and age-appropriate information about sex, relationships, and consent empowers individuals to make informed choices. As education systems improve and adapt to include a broader spectrum of sexual and gender identities, future generations will be better equipped to navigate their intimate lives with confidence and respect for themselves and others.

Conclusion

The future of intimacy and eroticism is one of transformation and possibility. Technological advancements, shifting societal norms, and a greater emphasis on mental health and education are all shaping a new landscape where people can explore their desires more freely and authentically. As we move forward, embracing diversity, fostering open communication, and prioritizing ethical and sustainable practices will be key to creating a more inclusive and fulfilling world of intimacy.